Mohd N. Zakaria
Joav Merrick
Editors

Public Health

Audiology Research in Malaysia

nova
Medicine & Health
New York

DOI: https://doi.org/10.52305/FHXB6681

Library of Congress Cataloging-in-Publication Data

ISBN: 979-8-89530-577-5 (Hardcover)
ISBN: 979-8-89530-663-5 (eBook)

Published by Nova Science Publishers, Inc. † New York

Contents

Introduction 1

Chapter 1 **Audiology: An emerging profession in Malaysia** 3
Mohd N Zakaria and Joav Merrick

Section one: **Public health and audiology** 9

Chapter 2 **Listening difficulties in children with auditory processing disorder (APD) in noisy and reverberant environments** 11
Mohd Z Azali, Wan NW Mohamad, Nashrah Maamor, Maziah Romli and Mohd N Zakaria

Chapter 3 **The performance of the auditory steady state response (ASSR) test in the prediction of behavioural hearing thresholds** 19
Muhammad SI Anual, Nik AN Othman, Mohd FN Rashid, Mahamad A Awang, Wan NW Mohamad and Mohd N Zakaria

Chapter 4 **Aided cortical auditory evoked potential (CAEP) outcomes in hearing-impaired children** 31
Nurnazeha Isnan, Rosninda Abdullah, Mohd FN Rashid, Nik AN Othman, Wan NW Mohamad, Nashrah Maamor and Mohd N Zakaria

Chapter 5 **Understanding the neural processing of cochlear implant users: Insights from cortical auditory evoked potential (CAEP) findings**..................................41
Rosninda Abdullah, Noor AA Wahab, Nashrah Maamor, Nik AN Othman, Basyariatul F Othman and Mohd N Zakaria

Chapter 6 **Managing patients with tinnitus: The potential role of teleaudiology**.................................53
Shameera Nizamuddin, Mohd N Zakaria, Mohd FN Rashid, Wan SW Husain and Wan NW Mohamad

Chapter 7 **Exploring the neural basis of tinnitus: Insights into auditory processing mechanisms from auditory brainstem response (ABR) studies** 63
Shamhana A Yusri, Mohd N Zakaria, Nik AN Othman, Cheu L Aw and Wan NW Mohamad

Section two: **Hearing**...73

Chapter 8 **Cervical vestibular evoked myogenic potential (VEMP) to wide-band chirp and tone burst stimuli: A comparative analysis** 75
Mohd N Zakaria, Wan NW Mohamad and Zuraida Zainun

Chapter 9 **Exploring cervical vestibular evoked myogenic potential (VEMP) when recorded with downward chirp stimuli of different frequency ranges**..85
Athar MR Abdallatif, Wan NW Mohamad, Rosdan Salim and Mohd N Zakaria

Chapter 10 **The influence of transducer type on the normative values in the sensorineural acuity level (SAL) test** 95
Rosdan Salim, Mahamad A Awang, Nik AN Othman, Mohd FN Rashid and Mohd N Zakaria

Chapter 11 **Laryngeal high-speed videoendoscopy: Vocal fold vibratory characteristics of normal speakers** 105
Khairy Anuar Mohd Khairuddin, Kartini Ahmad, Hasherah Mohd Ibrahim and Yuling Yan

Chapter 12 **The effect of complex auditory stimulations on auditory brainstem response (ABR) in healthy adults** 121
Noor AA Wahab, Suzaily Wahab, Nashrah Maamor, Wan NW Mohamad and Mohd N Zakaria

Chapter 13 **Assessing the auditory brainstem function in patients with schizophrenia: An acoustic reflex study** 129
Noor AA Wahab, Suzaily Wahab, Rafidah Mazlan, Mahamad A Awang and Mohd N Zakaria

Chapter 14 **Understanding the neural processing of hearing-impaired children: An aided cortical auditory evoked potential (CAEP) study** 139
Nurnazeha Isnan, Rosninda Abdullah, Nik AN Othman, Wan NW Mohamad, Nashrah Maamor and Mohd N Zakaria

Section three: **Miscellaneous issues** 149

Chapter 15 **Pure tone audiometry (PTA) and cross-hearing** 151
Mohd N Zakaria, Nik AN Othman, Cheu L Aw, Mohd FN Rashid, Mahamad A Awang, Wan NW Mohamad and Rafidah Mazlan

Chapter 16 **The effect of electrode montage on the aided cortical auditory evoked potential (CAEP)** 161
Nurnazeha Isnan, Rosninda Abdullah, Nik AN Othman, Wan NW Mohamad, Nashrah Maamor and Mohd N Zakaria

Chapter 17 **Pure tone audiometry (PTA) and diagnosing hearing problems** 171
Mohd N Zakaria

Chapter 18 **Understanding the relationship between cochlear implant (CI) mapping and cortical auditory evoked potential (CAEP)** 179
Rosninda Abdullah, Noor AA Wahab, Nashrah Maamor, Nik AN Othman, Basyariatul F Othman and Mohd N Zakaria

Chapter 19 **Treatment options for a baby with Luc's abscess** 189
Mohamad N Salleh, Mohd N Zakaria and Nik AN Othman

Chapter 20 **Diagnosing Meniere's disease with pure tone audiometry** 197
Mohd N Zakaria, Wan NW Mohamad, Cheu L Aw, Mohd FN Rashid, Mahamad A Awang and Marniza Omar

Chapter 21 **The audiometric Weber test versus the tuning fork Weber test for hearing diagnosis: Which one is better?** 205
Mohd N Zakaria

Chapter 22 **The clinical value of the subjective visual vertical (SVV) test with a complex visual image** 213
Rosdan Salim, Nurul SM Sakeri, Saiful A Jamaluddin, Nor HA Wahat and Mohd N Zakaria

Section four: **Acknowledgments**........221

Chapter 23 **About the Editors**........223

Chapter 24 **About the Audiology Programme, School of Health Sciences, Universiti Sains Malaysia, Kelantan, Malaysia**........225

Chapter 25 **About the National Institute of Child Health and Human Development in Israel**........229

Section five: **Index**........233

Index 235

Introduction

Chapter 1

Audiology: An emerging profession in Malaysia

Mohd N Zakaria[1], PhD
and Joav Merrick[2-4], MD, MMedSci, DMSc

[1]Audiology Programme, School of Health Sciences, Universiti Sains Malaysia, Kelantan, Malaysia
[2]Division of Pediatrics, Hadassah Hebrew University Medical Center, Israel
[3]Kentucky Children's Hospital, University of Kentucky, Lexington, United States of America
[4]Center for Healthy Development, School of Public Health, Georgia State University, Atlanta, United States of America

Abstract

The audiology education started late in Malaysia compared to other countries, but this clinical profession has shown remarkable and significant growth over the years. This growth is evident in the expanding number of audiology programs in Malaysian universities, the rising enrolment of students pursuing audiology degrees and the growing presence of audiologists in healthcare settings across the country. Furthermore, advancements in audiological research and the adoption of cutting-edge diagnostic and therapeutic technologies have also contributed to the profession's progress. As the field continues to evolve along with continuous research efforts, it is likely that audiology will play an even more vital role in addressing the needs of Malaysians in the years to come. In this book we will provide you with research and clinical experience from this emerging field.

In: Public Health: Audiology Research in Malaysia
Editors: Mohd N. Zakaria and Joav Merrick
ISBN: 979-8-89530-577-5

Introduction

Audiology plays a critical role in the healthcare system, providing essential services for individuals with hearing loss, tinnitus, vestibular disorders, and related conditions (1-3). Given the high prevalence of these issues across various age groups, the expertise of audiologists is indispensable. In Malaysia, the field of audiology has a relatively recent history, with the first professional education program launching in 1995. Herein, the National University of Malaysia took the lead in establishing audiology education in the country by introducing a 4-year Bachelor of Audiology degree. This program laid the foundation for audiology education nationally. Both the International Islamic University Malaysia and Universiti Sains Malaysia have since followed this precedent, developing their own undergraduate audiology degrees. The collective aim of these institutions is to ensure a supply of qualified audiologists to serve all regions of Malaysia. Importantly, the audiology programs provided by the aforementioned institutions are accredited and closely monitored by the Malaysian Qualification Agency (MQA) to ensure that audiology graduates possess the necessary knowledge and clinical competency. The implementation of outcome-based education ensures all graduates are impeccably equipped to meet the demands of their chosen industries upon entering the workforce (4).

Presently

At present, the field of audiology comprises approximately 800 practitioners across diverse sectors throughout the nation. The profession of audiology encompasses a wide and varied scope of practice. This includes, but is not limited to, diagnostic audiology, rehabilitative audiology, industrial audiology, and others. It is noteworthy that the majority of audiologists secure employment within hospital settings. Recent advancements in hearing amplification technologies have even unequivocally demonstrated the imperative need for audiologists. In year 2006, an audiology taskforce was established nationally to monitor audiological services throughout Malaysia. However, based on the ratio of audiologists to patients (considering a population of 32 million Malaysians), the number of audiologists in Malaysia is still insufficient. Therefore, increasing the number of audiologists and conducting relevant, impactful research is imperative to enhance the quality of audiological procedures and interventions.

Research

In terms of research, the three Malaysian universities collectively host around 30 active audiology researchers. While their research concentrations differ substantially, they encompass all areas of audiology. Over the years, they have generated numerous high-impact findings in the fields of diagnostic audiology, auditory evoked potential, hearing amplification, auditory rehabilitation, tinnitus, and vestibular. Many research outcomes and clinical experiences have been disseminated through peer-reviewed, indexed journals. Among others, Rafidah Mazlan and her colleagues at the National University of Malaysia have been at the forefront of research into the application of wideband tympanometry in infants (5, 6). In order to ameliorate the lives of elderly individuals suffering from hearing loss, Siti Zamratol Maisarah Mukari and her team have developed and validated a novel computer-based auditory training program (7, 8). It is recognized that patients experiencing auditory hallucinations may also have comorbid, yet undiagnosed, auditory disorders. Accordingly, Noor Alaudin Abdul Wahab and his colleagues have conducted innovative research into the audiological profiles of individuals with schizophrenia, employing advanced assessment techniques (9, 10). Research at the International Islamic University Malaysia, under the direction of Ahmad Aidil Arafat Dzulkarnain, has placed a significant emphasis on the fundamental aspects of chirp-evoked auditory brainstem response (ABR) (11, 12).

Acknowledging the limitations of pure tone audiometry in detecting certain auditory dysfunctions, there is a clear need to have speech audiometry assessments validated in the Malay version. In light of this, Saiful Adli Jamaluddin and his research team members have meticulously undertaken a sequence of investigations to develop and validate diverse speech assessments in the Malay language for utilization within clinical contexts (13, 14). On the other hand, a significant proportion of research articles pertaining to vestibular and tinnitus studies emanate from researchers at the Universiti Sains Malaysia. Recognizing the critical importance of accurate assessments and effective treatments for patients suffering from tinnitus and vestibular disorders, Mohd Normani Zakaria and his esteemed colleagues have dedicated their research to making a meaningful impact in these fields (15-19). Their study outcomes have shed new light on the complex nature of these conditions, paving the way for advancements in diagnosis, management, and ultimately, improving the quality of life for countless individuals affected by tinnitus and vestibular disorders. Specifically, the clinical efficacy of customized sound therapy and psychoaudiological intervention in treating those with tinnitus has been extensively researched (15-17).

Given the clinical significance, the efficacy of a home-based vestibular rehabilitation technique has been investigated, leading to its widespread adoption by numerous vestibular centres throughout Malaysia (18, 19). Furthermore, researchers at the Universiti Sains Malaysia have also studied the applications of advanced auditory evoked potentials including speech-evoked ABR and cortical auditory evoked potential (CAEP) evoked electrically and acoustically among children with hearing aids and cochlear implants (20-22). As technology continues to advance and shape the healthcare landscape, innovations in telemedicine are expanding access to vital services for patients around the world. In line with the recent development in the medical field, a team of researchers led by Mohd Fadzil Nor Rashid and his colleagues have studied the perception, usability, and applicability of teleaudiology in Malaysia (23, 24). Their work aims to understand how this emerging field can overcome traditional barriers to audiological care, improving outcomes for those in need.

References

[1] Goulios H, Patuzzi RB. Audiology education and practice from an international perspective. Int J Audiol 2008;47(10):647-64.

[2] Radzi AM, Zakaria MN, Ahmad A. Self-esteem, life satisfaction, and quality of life among audiology students. Int J Disabil Dev Educ 2024 May 13. doi: 10.1080/1034912X.2024.2355346.

[3] Romli M, Wan Mohamad WN, Awang MA, Aw CL, Zakaria MN. The clinical value of bilateral bone conduction testing in hearing diagnosis. Indian J Otol 2020;26(3):182-5.

[4] Davis MH. Outcome-based education. J Vet Med Educ 2003;30(3):258-63.

[5] Wali HA, Mazlan R, Kei J. Pressurized wideband absorbance findings in healthy neonates: A preliminary study. J Speech Lang Hear Res 2017;60(10):2965-73.

[6] Wali HA, Mazlan R, Kei J. A longitudinal analysis of pressurized wideband absorbance measures in healthy young infants. Ear Hear 2019;40(5):1233-41.

[7] Bani NH, Maamor N, Mukari SZM, Ishak WS, Chellappan K. Usability and acceptance of a computer-based auditory training among older adults in Malaysia. Int J Disabil Hum Dev 2019;18(3):345-54.

[8] Bani NH, Maamor N, Mukari SZM, Ishak WS, Chellappan K. Development of Malay sentence materials in speech-in-noise training for adults. Int J Disabil Hum Dev 2019;18(3):325-32.

[9] Wahab S, Zakaria MN, Sidek D, Abdul Rahman AH, Shah SA, Abdul Wahab NA. Evaluation of auditory hallucinations in patients with schizophrenia: A validation study of the Malay version of Psychotic Symptom Rating Scales (PSYRATS). Psychiatry Res 2015;228(3):462-7.

[10] Abdul Wahab NA, Wahab S, Abdul Rahman AH, Sidek D, Zakaria MN. The hyperactivity of efferent auditory system in patients with schizophrenia: A transient evoked otoacoustic emissions study. Psychiatry Investig 2016;13(1):82-8.

[11] Dzulkarnain AAA, Shahrudin FA, Jamal FN, Marzuki MN, Mazlan MNS. Effects of stimulus repetition rates on the auditory brainstem response to level-specific CE-chirp in normal-hearing adults. Am J Audiol 2020;29(4):838-50.

[12] Dzulkarnain AAA, Rahed BAM, Shahrudin FA, Jamal FN, Zakaria MN. Effects of ambient acoustic noise on auditory brainstem response to level-specific chirp and click stimuli in normal-hearing adults. J Audiol Otol 2022;26(4):182-91.

[13] Zakaria NA, Jamaluddin SA, Wan Ahmad WAS, O'Beirne GA, Zulkeflee NA, Abd Razak A. The development of paediatric Malay matrix sentence test (PaedMalayMST) materials through the construction of a paediatric Malay corpus. J Mod Lang 2022;32(2):1-16.

[14] Salahuddin NB, Jamaluddin SA, Lamri M, Ali Hanafiah N, Sidek D. Can articulation index better estimate speech intelligibility on adult cochlear implant users compared to aided pure tone thresholds? Int J Allied Health Sci 2023;7(5): 1-9.

[15] Wan Suhailah WH, Mohd Normani Z, Nik Adilah NO, Azizah O, Aw CL, Zuraida Z. The effectiveness of psychological interventions among tinnitus sufferers: A review. Med J Malaysia 2015;70(3):188-97.

[16] Zakaria MN. The effectiveness of sound therapy in treating patients with mild and severe tinnitus. Int J Disabil Hum Dev 2020;19(2):215-9.

[17] Wong JW, Wan Mohamad WN, Wan Husain WS, Zakaria MN. The tinnitus suppressive effect: Comparisons between three types of maskers. Int J Disabil Hum Dev 2020;19(1):21-6.

[18] Bayat A, Pourbakht A, Saki N, Zainun Z, Nikakhlagh S, Mirmomeni G. Vestibular rehabilitation outcomes in the elderly with chronic vestibular dysfunction. Iran Red Crescent Med J 2012;14(11):705-8.

[19] Teh CS, Abdullah NA, Kamaruddin NR, Mohd Judi KB, Fadzilah I, Zainun Z, et al. Home-based vestibular rehabilitation: A feasible and effective therapy for persistent postural perceptual dizziness (a pilot study). Ann Otol Rhinol Laryngol 2023;132(5):566-77.

[20] Zakaria MN, Jalaei B, Aw CL, Sidek D. Are speech-evoked auditory brainstem response (speech-ABR) outcomes influenced by ethnicity? Neurol Sci 2016;37(6):943-8.

[21] Jalaei B, Azmi MHAM, Zakaria MN. Gender differences in binaural speech-evoked auditory brainstem response: are they clinically significant? Braz J Otorhinolaryngol 2019;85(4):486-93.

[22] Mukari SZS, Umat C, Chan SC, Ali A, Maamor N, Zakaria MN. Effects of age and type of stimulus on the cortical auditory evoked potential in healthy Malaysian children. J Audiol Otol 2020;24(1):35-9.
[23] Quar TK, Rashid MFN, Rosdi MYM, Ishak WS, Chong FY. Impact of the COVID-19 pandemic on individuals with hearing loss and audiology practice in a developing country. Am J Audiol 2023;32(1):59-69.
[24] Rashid MFN, Maamor N, Foong Yen C, Kar QT. Development of teleaudiology service in special education service centre in malaysia: lessons learned. J Adv Res Appl Sci Eng Technol 2024;34(1):289-98.

Section one: Public health and audiology

Chapter 2

Listening difficulties in children with auditory processing disorder (APD) in noisy and reverberant environments

Mohd Z Azali[1], BSc
Wan NW Mohamad[1], PhD
Nashrah Maamor[2], PhD
Maziah Romli[1], MSc
and Mohd N Zakaria[1], PhD

[1]Audiology Programme, School of Health Sciences, Universiti Sains Malaysia, Kelantan, Malaysia
[2] Centre for Ear, Hearing and Speech, Faculty of Health Sciences, Universiti Kebangsaan Malaysia, Kuala Lumpur, Malaysia

Abstract

It has been reported that, despite having normal hearing sensitivity, some children have hearing difficulties in school settings, i.e., in noisy and reverberant classrooms. This complex condition is known as auditory processing disorder (APD), and it is believed to occur due to disruptions within the central auditory nervous system (CANS). Due to its complexity, the gold standard test for diagnosing APD is not yet available universally. Since children who are at risk for having APD may show more than one auditory difficulty, it is agreeable that a test battery approach is required. Several guidelines have been proposed to provide researchers and clinicians with essential information regarding how to assess, diagnose, and manage children with APD. Nevertheless, little is known about the impact of reverberation on speech perception in children

In: Public Health: Audiology Research in Malaysia
Editors: Mohd N. Zakaria and Joav Merrick
ISBN: 979-8-89530-577-5

with APD. In this chapter, the fundamental information of APD is described accordingly, including the common auditory difficulties faced by APD children, as well as the important issues in APD assessments. The emphasis is made on the effect of noise and reverberation on speech intelligibility in individuals with auditory disorders. Based on the existing accumulated evidence, more research efforts are required to provide better information regarding the specific difficulties faced by children with APD in their real-life listening situations in noisy and reverberant classrooms. Developing and validating a simple APD screening tool employing noise and reverberation elements for school children can be the next step.

Introduction

Hearing is an important human sense that enables people to enjoy communication in their daily lives. When a sound reaches the external ear, it is then transmitted to the middle ear and the inner ear. This peripheral auditory system is important to amplify and analyse the acoustic features of the sound (1). Subsequently, the auditory nerve is responsible for transmitting the auditory information (in the form of electrical impulses) to the central auditory nervous system (CANS) (i.e., brainstem, subcortical and cortical regions) for further processing (2).

For children, having intact hearing abilities is crucial to ensuring normal speech and language skills, good academic performance, and adequate psychosocial skills. In this regard, those with hearing loss must be diagnosed and treated in a timely manner to minimize the negative consequences of hearing loss (1, 3). In cases of peripheral hearing loss, various subjective and objective audiological tests are available in clinical settings to aid in the diagnosis of hearing loss (4-11). Pure tone audiometry (PTA) is a subjective audiological test that is typically conducted to provide information on the severity of hearing loss and the type of hearing loss for both ears (4). In this assessment, hearing thresholds (i.e., the softest sounds that are heard by an individual) are determined in a quiet soundproof room. As reported elsewhere, hearing thresholds that are equal to or less than 20 dB HL are considered normal (1). Speech audiometry is another subjective test conducted to measure speech perception in a quiet environment, as well to verify PTA results (1). If the PTA results are unreliable or questionable, objective audiological tests such as otoacoustic emission (OAE), auditory brainstem response (ABR), auditory steady state response (ASSR) and cortical auditory evoked potential

(CAEP) can be the next options (7-11). By performing these electrophysiological tests, hearing thresholds can be estimated appropriately (1).

It is evident that some children have hearing difficulties in school settings (12, 13). In particular, they could not hear well conversations and teachers' instructions in noisy and echoic classrooms. Interestingly, their audiological test results can be normal (i.e., hearing thresholds ≤ 20 dB HL in PTA and 100% score in speech audiometry). This condition is known as auditory processing disorder (APD) and is believed to occur due to CANS dysfunctions (2, 12, 13).

Characteristics of auditory processing disorder (APD)

By definition, APD is a specific disorder affecting the processing of auditory information within the CANS (12). Its prevalence is estimated to be around 5%-10% among the general population (2, 14, 15). Children with APD are at risk for having difficulties listening and learning despite having normal hearing sensitivity (12, 13). Specifically, they may show difficulties in auditory localization, auditory discrimination, auditory pattern recognition, temporal aspects of audition (including resolution, masking, integration, and ordering), understanding speech with competing acoustic signals, as well as when acoustic signals are degraded (12, 13, 16). APD can also impede communication, social, emotional, and work elements of life. Furthermore, if untreated, it can have a negative impact on an individual's psychological states (self-esteem, anxiety, and depression), and its symptoms can last into adulthood (17).

There have been ongoing debates regarding the best approach to assess, diagnose, and treat individuals with APD (12, 16, 17). Currently, the gold standard test for assessing APD is not yet available. This situation is further complicated by its common co-morbidity with other conditions (e.g., attention deficit disorder, speech and language problems, learning disabilities, etc.) (12, 13). Due to the fact that children with APD have normal hearing thresholds and excellent speech discrimination scores when tested in a quiet situation but show the respective symptoms in non-optimum environments, the APD tests must be designed to be "challenging" and "difficult" (13). For example, in the auditory figure ground (AFG) test, a listener is required to repeat words or sentences that are presented at a supra-threshold level (e.g., 65 dB HL) in the presence of competing background noise (12). Sensibly, since the noise is also present (which mimics the real-life situation in the classrooms), children with APD may show poor scores (even though their speech scores in quiet are excellent). Likewise, in the competing words (CW) test, the listener is instructed to repeat all words that he or she hears (i.e., two words to each ear simultaneously). Poor results indicate some abnormality at the cortical level (related to the binaural integration function) (12).

Since APD children may show multiple auditory difficulties, a test battery approach has been recommended (as a single test is not adequate to properly diagnose APD) (12, 16, 17). However, the duration of testing must also be appropriate (i.e., having too many tests can be problematic). In line with this, in 1996, the American Speech-Hearing Association (ASHA) task force on APD was initiated to propose the types of APD tests and the minimum number of tests to be used when assessing those who are at risk for having APD (12). Subsequent amendments were made in 2001 based on the current research findings (16). In particular, they recommended that an APD test battery should include at least 4 subtests that consist of auditory pattern/temporal ordering tasks, monaural separation/closure tasks, binaural separation tasks and binaural integration tasks (16). In 2017, a group of European APD experts reported a baseline European APD consensus (17). This guideline was developed with the aim of providing the respective APD researchers and clinicians with the latest information on how to properly assess and manage individuals with APD. Nevertheless, no specific recommendation was made regarding the types of APD tests to be used, and the issue of not having the gold standard test for evaluating APD remains unresolved.

The effects of noise and reverberation on speech perception

As mentioned earlier, children with APD may show their symptoms in non-optimum listening environments (e.g., noisy and reverberant classrooms). As such, to properly diagnose this disorder, test materials employing noise and reverberation elements can be advantageous. In a typical classroom, when someone speaks, his/her voice can travel directly to the listeners and also hit hard surfaces, causing sound reflections. Reverberation is the persistence of echo (i.e., reflected sounds) after the sound source has been terminated. It is typically described in terms of its reverberation time, i.e., the time taken for the sound intensity level in a room to drop by 60 dB from its initial level. The reverberation time is dependent on the size and the acoustical features of the room, and for typical classrooms (with no absorbent materials for the wall, floor, or ceiling), it can be as high as 2 seconds (18,19). The recommended upper limit of the reverberation time considered to be optimum is 0.6 seconds (20-22). In this regard, longer reverberation times can potentially affect the speech intelligibility (18).

Many studies have shown that individuals with auditory disorders have problems to perceive speech sounds in reverberant rooms (22-25). The addition of higher noise levels in the classrooms further complicates the listening situation (22-24). The guideline provided by the ASHA task force on APD also specifically stated that children with APD may have problems listening to degraded acoustic signals (12,16). Nevertheless, it is worth noting that not many studies have been conducted to specifically evaluate the impacts of noise and reverberation on speech perception in children with APD. Most of the studies investigated the effects of noise and reverberation among healthy children, those with peripheral hearing loss, and elderly adults (22-26).

In a classroom context, it is difficult to have separate acoustic conditions, and most of the time the acoustic conditions occur in their combination (noise plus reverberation) (22). School children, especially those who have auditory processing problems, are potentially affected by these classroom acoustic conditions. The decibel signal to noise ratio (dB SNR), which is 7 dB and above, is necessary for children with hearing loss to understand speech sounds relative to normal children (i.e., 4 dB and above), especially in the echoic room settings. For educational purposes, a good classroom acoustic should have an SNR of at least 15 dB and a reverberation time between 0.4 and 0.6 seconds (22). Yet, given the nature of the classroom settings, which are susceptible to various noise and echo sources, this is challenging to accomplish.

In line with this, Johnson conducted a study to assess the effects of reverberation, noise, and their combination on listeners' identification of consonants and vowels in naturally produced nonsense syllables (27). Participants were normally hearing children and adults aged from 6 to 30 years (n = 80). The stimuli were presented at different sensation levels and in different listening conditions (i.e., quiet, reverberation, noise, and reverberation plus noise). The results revealed that the participants performed better in vowel identification and at the highest sensation level (i.e., 50 dB SL). The performance of children was inferior to that of adults, particularly in consonant identification and in complex listening conditions. It was then concluded that for different components of the speech signals, the ability to distinguish speech sounds in reverberation and noise would achieve adult-like levels of performance at different ages (27).

More recently, Cameron and her colleagues developed an assessment tool, known as the Language-Independent Speech in Noise and Reverberation test (LISiNaR), aiming to measure the ability of individuals listening functions when noise and reverberation are present (28). Additionally, they also wanted to investigate how participants from different language backgrounds performed in the auditory processing assessment. Pseudo-words were used as targets and distractors (presented with headphones), and the listening environment was simulated using reverberant and anechoic head-related transfer functions. The results gathered from healthy adult participants (aged 18-35 years) who were native speakers of Australian (n = 24), Canadian (n = 25), and non-native English speakers (n = 34) revealed no language effect in the tool's usage. The effect of reverberation on speech reception threshold in noise was reasonably small (i.e., 5 dB).

Future directions

APD is a complex and heterogeneous condition that requires specialised assessments and treatments by the respective clinical experts. Even though various APD assessments have been developed and studied accordingly, the search for a better test is still ongoing (as the gold standard test for diagnosing APD is not yet available). In this regard, having a simple and rapid APD screening test employing noise and reverberation elements (to mimic the real-life classroom environments) can be beneficial for identifying APD among school children in a timely manner. In a country such as Malaysia, children aged 4–6 years will be cultivated into positive school readiness attitudes through informal education programmes before entering the formal school system (29). Around seven years of age, the children will be entering the real world of education, where they will learn in a formal education system involving skills in reading, writing, and arithmetic, as well as other values across the curriculum (30). Herein, it is important to identify any problems that can impair the learning process so that proper interventions can be applied accordingly. One of the elements that is essential in the learning process is listening, and identifying listening problems (i.e., due to APD) is therefore imperative. Conducting further research on this aspect will also pave the way for a better understanding of the specific effects of noise and reverberation on speech perception in children with APD.

Acknowledgments

This chapter was part of a study funded by the Short Term Grant of Universiti Sains Malaysia with Project Code: 304/PPSK/6315420.

References

[1] Katz J, Chasin M, English K, Hood L, Tillery KL. Handbook of clinical audiology. Philadelphia, PA: Lippincott Williams Wilkins, 2015.

[2] Chermak GD, Musiek FE. Central auditory processing disorders: new perspectives. San Diego, CA: Singular Publishing Group, 1997.

[3] Yoshinaga-Itano C. Benefits of early intervention for children with hearing loss. Otolaryngol Clin North Am 1999;32(6):1089-102.

[4] Wan Mohamad WN, Romli M, Awang MA, Abdullah R, Lih AC, Zakaria MN. The presence of unusual bone conduction thresholds in pure tone audiometry. Indian J Otol 2020;26(1):54-7.

[5] Romli M, Wan Mohamad WN, Awang MA, Aw CL, Zakaria MN. The clinical value of bilateral bone conduction testing in hearing diagnosis. Indian J Otol 2020;26(3):182-5.

[6] Lih AC, Zakaria MN, Mohamad RA, Nor Rashid MF. Effects of ethnicity and gender on the middle ear function in Asian adults. Indian J Otol 2017;23(2):94-7.

[7] Abdul Wahab NA, Wahab S, Abdul Rahman AH, Sidek D, Zakaria MN. The hyperactivity of efferent auditory system in patients with schizophrenia: a transient evoked otoacoustic emissions study. Psychiatry Investig 2016;13(1):82-8.

[8] Zakaria MN, Jalaei B, Wahab NA. Gender and modulation frequency effects on auditory steady state response (ASSR) thresholds. Eur Arch Otorhinolaryngol 2016;273(2):349-54.

[9] Zakaria MN, Jalaei B, Aw CL, Sidek D. Are speech-evoked auditory brainstem response (speech-ABR) outcomes influenced by ethnicity? Neurol Sci 2016;37(6):943-8.

[10] Jalaei B, Zakaria MN, Mohd Azmi MH, Nik Othman NA, Sidek D. Gender disparities in speech-evoked auditory brainstem response in healthy Adults. Ann Otol Rhinol Laryngol 2017;126(4):290-5.

[11] Mukari SZS, Umat C, Chan SC, Ali A, Maamor N, Zakaria MN. Effects of age and type of stimulus on the cortical auditory evoked potential in healthy Malaysian children. J Audiol Otol 2020;24(1):35-9.

[12] American Speech-Language-Hearing Association. Central auditory processing: current status of research and implications for clinical practice. Am J Audiol 1996;5(2):41-54.

[13] Zakaria MN. Auditory localization in subjects with central auditory processing disorders. Doctoral dissertation. Perth: The University of Western Australia, 2007.

[14] Bamiou DE, Musiek FE, Luxon LM. Aetiology and clinical presentations of auditory processing disorders-a review. Arch Dis Child 2001;85(5):361-5.

[15] Hind SE, Haines-Bazrafshan R, Benton CL, Brassington W, Towle B, Moore DR. Prevalence of clinical referrals having hearing thresholds within normal limits. Int J Audiol 2011;50(10):708-16.

[16] Schow RL, Seikel JA, Chermak GD, Berent M. Central auditory processes and test measures: ASHA 1996 revisited. Am J Audiol 2000;9(2):63-8.

[17] Iliadou VV, Ptok M, Grech H, Pedersen ER, Brechmann A, Deggouj N, et al. A European perspective on auditory processing disorder-current knowledge and future research focus. Front Neurol 2017;8:622.

[18] Rabelo AT, Santos JN, Oliveira RC, Magalhães Mde C. Effect of classroom acoustics on the speech intelligibility of students. Codas 2014;26(5):360-6.

[19] Tong YG, Md Amin ND, Othman MH, Abas NH, Ewon U, Mohd Zaim MAZ, et al. Assessments of acoustical performance of classrooms and teachers' acoustical comfort in the school environment – a case study. Int J Integr Eng 2022;14(6):406-14.

[20] Bistafa SR, Bradley JS. Optimum acoustical conditions for speech intelligibility in classrooms. Noise Vib Worldw 2000;31(9):12-7.

[21] Zannin PHT, Marcon CR. Objective and subjective evaluation of the acoustic comfort in classrooms. Appl Ergon 2007;38(5):675-80.

[22] Nelson PB, Soli S. Acoustical barriers to learning: children at risk in every classroom. Lang Speech Hear Serv Sch 2000;31(4):356-61.

[23] Schepker H, Haeder K, Rennies J, Holube I. Perceived listening effort and speech intelligibility in reverberation and noise for hearing-impaired listeners. Int J Audiol 2016;55(12):738-47.

[24] George EL, Goverts ST, Festen JM, Houtgast T. Measuring the effects of reverberation and noise on sentence intelligibility for hearing-impaired listeners. J Speech Lang Hear Res 2010;53(6):1429-39.

[25] Halling DC, Humes LE. Factors affecting the recognition of reverberant speech by elderly listeners. J Speech Lang Hear Res 2000;43(2):414-31.

[26] Gheller F, Lovo E, Arsie A, Bovo R. Classroom acoustics: listening problems in children. Build Acoust 2020;27(1):47-59.

[27] Johnson CE. Children's phoneme identification in reverberation and noise. J Speech Lang Hear Res 2000;43(1):144-57.

[28] Cameron S, Boyle C, Dillon H. The development of the Language-Independent Speech in Noise and Reverberation test (LISiNaR) and evaluation in listeners with English as a second language. Int J Audiol 2022;1-11.

[29] Rahmatullah B, Muhamad Rawai N, Mohamad Samuri S, Md Yassin S. Overview of early childhood care and education in Malaysia. Hung Educ Res J 2021;11(4):396-412.

[30] Dewi E, Selvarajoo J, Hassan Z, Mokhtar M. Resources distribution in Malaysian education system. Int J Innov Educ Res 2014;2(10):177-84.

Chapter 3

The performance of the auditory steady state response (ASSR) test in the prediction of behavioural hearing thresholds

Muhammad SI Anual[1], BSc
Nik AN Othman[2], MMed
Mohd FN Rashid[1], PhD
Mahamad A Awang[1], MClinAud
Wan NW Mohamad[1], PhD
and Mohd N Zakaria[1], PhD
[1]Audiology Programme, School of Health Sciences, Universiti Sains Malaysia, Kelantan, Malaysia
[2]Department of Otorhinolaryngology, School of Medical Sciences, Universiti Sains Malaysia, Kelantan, Malaysia

Abstract

It is crucial for children to have normal speech, language, and communication abilities. This is made possible if they have an intact hearing function. In this regard, any potential hearing loss should be detected earlier so that an appropriate intervention can take place in a timely manner. Nevertheless, getting valid and reliable hearing information from children can be challenging. The application of objective hearing tests is useful so that hearing thresholds can be estimated accordingly (and "cooperation" from the patients is not needed). Among others, auditory steady state response (ASSR) has been gaining attention among researchers and clinicians. In this chapter, the advantages of ASSR as an objective test for estimating hearing thresholds

In: Public Health: Audiology Research in Malaysia
Editors: Mohd N. Zakaria and Joav Merrick
ISBN: 979-8-89530-577-5

are highlighted accordingly, including the use of automated signal detection algorithms and optimized chirp stimuli. The performance of ASSR in predicting behavioural thresholds in normal and hearing-impaired individuals is described as intended. In addition, factors that affect the accuracy of ASSR are also discussed. Based on the available evidence, more studies are needed to further improve the capability of ASSR in estimating behavioural thresholds. The next step could be to conduct research on how machine learning can be used to improve ASSR accuracy.

Introduction

Hearing is one of the valuable senses that enables people to enjoy communication in their daily lives. If the auditory is compromised, the affected individuals may complain of hearing loss and related disorders (1-5). Hearing loss is in fact a prevalent medical condition, with 466 million people are estimated to have some form of hearing loss (and this number is expected to rise to more than 700 million by 2050) (6). As reported elsewhere (7,8), hearing loss can have a significant impact on one's quality of life, causing anxiety, depression, social isolation and others. Hence, identifying and managing hearing loss in a timely manner is essential to minimize the negative effects of hearing loss, leading to improved quality of life and communication.

In clinical settings, various hearing tests are carried out to appropriately diagnose the severity of hearing loss and the type of hearing loss among adults and paediatric patients (9-15). Hearing healthcare professionals such as audiologists commonly use pure tone audiometry (PTA) for hearing diagnosis (1, 9). This subjective assessment has been regarded as the gold standard test for hearing assessment and represents how a person detects sounds at specific frequencies (1). However, due to its subjective nature, PTA results can be questionable in some cases. That is, it can be manipulated by malingerers and easily affected by attention and cooperation, particularly when assessing paediatric patients and those who are "difficult to test" (16, 17). Unreliable outcomes may lead to ineffective case management. Due to this, the capability to objectively evaluate the hearing function of patients whose behavioural thresholds are incomplete or questionable is of great interest.

To provide objective information on hearing thresholds, audiologists often utilize electrophysiological tests including auditory brainstem response (ABR), auditory steady state response (ASSR) and auditory middle latency response (AMLR) (11,16). Other tests such as electrocochleography

(ECochG) and cortical auditory evoked potential (CAEP) are typically carried out for site of lesion applications (15, 18). In these electrophysiological assessments, specific sounds are presented (via headphones or loudspeakers) and action potentials produced along the auditory system are recorded by surface electrodes (attached to specific locations of the head) while the patient is asleep or awake (with minimal body movements). The required waveforms are then analysed accordingly to estimate the behavioural thresholds (11).

Objective estimation of behavioural hearing thresholds by ASSR

Even though ECochG, ABR, AMLR and CAEP are able to provide objective information on the function of the auditory system, the waveform analysis is dependent on the knowledge, skill and experience of the tester. In this regard, "different" interpretations might be documented by newly graduated audiologists versus experienced audiologists (11). Furthermore, some ABR results can be difficult to analyse and require in-depth discussions among the experts (19, 20). The ASSR testing, on the other hand, utilizes a more convenient approach in the waveform analysis. That is, it employs specific signal detection algorithms and hearing thresholds are documented in a more objective manner (11, 13, 21, 22). Moreover, with the capability of estimating frequency-specific (500 Hz, 1000 Hz, 2000 Hz and 4000 Hz) hearing thresholds in both ears simultaneously, the testing time can be reduced tremendously (11).

Earlier studies on ASSR have confirmed that amplitude and/or frequency modulated tones are effective in evoking ASSR waveforms (23-26). These stimuli have been chosen to record ASSR, and several signal detection systems have been employed to objectively analyse the ASSR waveforms (21, 22, 25-27). When the ASSR device was first commercially developed in the 1990s, there were challenges with the automatic signal detection schemes (due to the lack of sufficient sensitivity to detect low-amplitude responses). The stimuli used and signal detection methods employed in the ASSR devices are rather complex (11). The response verification is typically accomplished through an automated statistical detection, comparing the response to the background noise within the electroencephalogram (EEG) spectrum. Some detection algorithms search for "coherence" in phase across segments (23, 25), while others evaluate the amplitude of the target frequency component in relation to the surrounding frequencies in the fast Fourier transform (FFT) (testing for statistical differences using an *F* test) (26). Some systems examine evidence of the responses through both phase and amplitude measurements (21, 22). Furthermore, recent advancements in the ASSR systems have incorporated a new detection algorithm capable of detecting amplitude and phase at up to 12 harmonics of the respective modulation frequency (27).

The ASSR testing can be used to assess the hearing status of adults and children, and the results can be integrated with the results of other tests to achieve an accurate hearing diagnosis. It can be recorded with a wide range of modulation frequencies (MFs), i.e., between 10 to 200 Hz (11). It is worth noting that the rate of MF may affect the signal-to-noise ratio (SNR) during the ASSR testing for infants and young children. As reported elsewhere, the SNR for ASSR in young children is better at higher MFs compared to lower MFs (28). Biological noise levels (EEG and myogenic activities) are reduced at higher MFs, whether in sedated or natural sleep condition. In this regard, the neural maturation is a dominant factor for this age group, and the immature auditory cortex causes difficulties in sustaining a rhythmic response at lower MFs. Therefore, it has been suggested that higher MFs (80 Hz or more) are better for the assessment of hearing thresholds in children, whereas lower MFs (40 Hz) are better when testing adults (28). When evoked with a 40 Hz MF, the ASSR is easily identified, and the amplitude obtained is relatively large (11). In fact, this response is present at intensity levels near behavioural thresholds and thus it could be used to predict hearing levels of an individual (13, 22). It is worth stating that the 40 Hz ASSR (or lower MFs) is contributed by neural generators at cortical levels (11, 24). On the other hand, at higher MFs (60 Hz and above), the response is generated predominantly by subcortical areas, especially the brainstem (11, 24).

The performance of ASSR in hearing thresholds estimation

Given its notable advantages, the ASSR test has become increasingly common in daily clinical practice for estimating hearing thresholds, especially in cases where other conventional methods may not be effective. Over recent years, many studies have examined the accuracy and effectiveness of ASSR in hearing thresholds estimation. Aimoni et al. (29) conducted a study to investigate the accuracy of ASSR in children with sensorineural hearing loss. The study outcomes highlighted the utility of ASSR in detecting hearing loss and estimating behavioural hearing thresholds. In a study conducted by

Tarawneh et al. (30), the ASSR and behavioural thresholds were compared in hearing-impaired adults. The study findings indeed support the accuracy and suitability of ASSR in daily clinical settings. Meanwhile, in a study by Aslam et al. (31), the accuracy of ASSR and ABR in predicting hearing thresholds was compared, and the effectiveness of ASSR in relation to ABR was highlighted from many perspectives.

There are numerous parameters such as hearing level, modulation frequency (MF), detection algorithm and type of stimulus which contribute to the efficiency of ASSR (32). Data from the literature have suggested that the amount of hearing loss significantly affects the difference between ASSR and PTA thresholds (11, 28, 33, 34). Generally, the discrepancy between behavioural and ASSR thresholds is less as hearing level increases and as carrier frequency (CF) increases (11, 33, 34). Furthermore, for 99% of the comparisons, the ASSR thresholds were found to be within 20 dB of the PTA thresholds, and for 82% of the comparisons, they were less than or equal to 10 dB (25). In line with this, better correlation and less disagreement are seen in patients with hearing loss than those with normal hearing (35-37). Owing to this, several studies have proposed regression formulae in order to predict behavioural thresholds (based on ASSR results), as well as "correction factors" (33, 35, 36, 38). The use of correction factors should sensibly provide better ASSR results (i.e., closer to the behavioural thresholds). Nevertheless, given that its thresholds may still overestimate PTA thresholds at some frequencies and underestimate PTA thresholds at other frequencies (even after the application of correction factors) (37, 39), the accuracy of ASSR may not improve as predicted.

The choice of MF is also critical when conducting the ASSR testing. Generally, low MFs produce more robust ASSR waveforms and better ASSR thresholds relative to high MFs (11, 13, 22, 40). Nevertheless, since the generators of ASSR are dependent on MF, high MFs (e.g., 90 Hz) are the choice when assessing infants and young children, as the ASSR waveforms are thought to be produced by the brainstem (11, 24), therefore less issues with maturity, sleeping, and sedation. For adults, even though both low and high MFs can be used, low MFs (e.g., 40 Hz) are a better option (13, 22, 40).

The type of stimulus has an impact on the robustness of ASSR waveforms. Even though amplitude and/or frequency modulated tones are good enough to elicit ASSR (11, 25, 26, 29), more recent studies have found that chirp stimuli are more efficient in evoking ASSR (13, 21, 22, 27, 31, 37). In particular, due to promising study outcomes, the narrowband CE-Chirp stimuli have been included in many commercially available ASSR devices (41). These stimuli were designed in such a way that they are able to compensate for the time delay related to the cochlear travelling wave (41, 42). By presenting lower-frequency stimuli earlier than higher-frequency sounds, this ensures that the stimuli arrive simultaneously along the entire basilar membrane, leading to synchronized firing of nerve fibres. This synchronization contributes to more precise ASSR results (43). As demonstrated elsewhere, the chirp stimuli have been found to produce ASSR thresholds closer to behavioural thresholds (with higher correlations) compared to other conventional stimuli (43, 44).

The applications of machine learning in clinical research

With the advancements in computing systems, the field of machine learning (ML) has emerged as a promising research domain for both theoretical and applied research (45). It is a subfield of artificial intelligence (AI) that explores how machines can learn a pattern from data to automatically perform a specific task (46). Depending on the availability of data and labels for training a model, these approaches can be categorized into two main branches, namely supervised and unsupervised. In supervised learning, the goal is to learn a mapping function that maps the input data to the labels. Subsequently, this learned function is utilized to predict labels for new and unseen data. On the other hand, unsupervised techniques explore the underlying structure or distribution in the data without labels. Semi-supervised learning comes into play when dealing with a substantial dataset, where only a portion of the data is labelled, while the majority remains unlabelled. ML has been applied in various fields to help with analysis and accuracy. In the field of medicine, the use of ML is becoming more prominent (47). It has enabled healthcare practitioners to reduce their manual workload and make more accurate judgments (48). Classifiers of ML such as discriminant analysis (DA), support vector machine (SVM), k-nearest neighbour (KNN), decision tree (DT) and artificial neural network (ANN) are commonly used in clinical studies (49). There are a number of studies conducted using ML algorithms to evaluate evoked responses, including ABR (45). Unfortunately, no study has evaluated the application of ML for hearing thresholds estimation using the ASSR. With this innovation, it can potentially open a new possibility for enhancing the accuracy of ASSR. It could have a substantial impact, leading to more precise diagnosis and tailored interventions.

Future directions

Hearing threshold estimation is a fundamental process used to assess an individual's hearing ability and detect any potential hearing loss or impairment. It is a method to determine the softest levels of sound that a person can hear across a range of frequencies. This information helps clinicians diagnose hearing impairment, assess the degree and type of hearing loss, and recommend appropriate interventions or treatments. An early detection of hearing loss is crucial, particularly for children, as it plays a critical role in the timely prescription of hearing aids. This allows children to acquire speech and language skills with the auditory stimulation provided by the hearing aids. Since it is an objective test, having an ASSR testing is particularly advantageous in assessing hearing thresholds of children and those whose behavioural thresholds are questionable. Nevertheless, more research efforts are required to further enhance the capability of ASSR in predicting behavioural thresholds. Among others, it is anticipated that the application of ML will be effective in enhancing the accuracy of ASSR in hearing diagnosis, as well as maintaining the quality and consistency of hearing test results. When efficiency and robustness are shown by the ASSR test, this will contribute to the improvement in intervention and management of the hearing-impaired population, as well as the provision of hearing healthcare services.

Acknowledgments

This chapter was part of a study funded by a research grant registered under Universiti Sains Malaysia with Project Code: 304/PPSK/6150272.

References

[1] Wan Mohamad WN, Romli M, Awang MA, Abdullah R, Lih AC, Zakaria MN. The presence of unusual bone conduction thresholds in pure tone audiometry. Indian J Otol 2020;26(1):54-7.

[2] Zuraida Z, Mohd Normani Z, Dinsuhaimi S, Zalina I, Geshina MS. Development of Malay version of vertigo symptom scale (MVVSS) for clinical use. Malaysian J Med Health Sci 2010;6(2):31-9.

[3] Wong JW, Wan Mohamad WN, Wan Husain WS, Zakaria MN. The tinnitus suppressive effect: Comparisons between three types of maskers. Int J Disabil Hum Dev 2020;19(1):21-6.

[4] Zakaria MN. The effectiveness of sound therapy in treating patients with mild and severe tinnitus. Int J Disabil Hum Dev 2020;19(2):215-9.

[5] Wahab S, Zakaria MN, Sidek D, Abdul Rahman AH, Shah SA, Abdul Wahab NA. Evaluation of auditory hallucinations in patients with schizophrenia: A validation study of the Malay version of Psychotic Symptom Rating Scales (PSYRATS). Psychiatry Res 2015;228(3):462-7.

[6] World Health Organization (WHO). Deafness and hearing loss, 2020. URL: https://www.who.int/news-room/fact-sheets/ detail/deafness-and-hearing-loss.

[7] Manrique-Huarte R, Calavia D, Huarte Irujo A, Girón L, Manrique-Rodríguez M. Treatment for hearing loss among the elderly: auditory outcomes and impact on quality of life. Audiol Neurootol 2016;21(Suppl 1):29-35.

[8] Yoshinaga-Itano C. Benefits of early intervention for children with hearing loss. Otolaryngol Clin North Am 1999;32(6):1089-102.

[9] Romli M, Wan Mohamad WN, Awang MA, Aw CL, Zakaria MN. The clinical value of bilateral bone conduction testing in hearing diagnosis. Indian J Otol 2020;26(3):182-5.

[10] Lih AC, Zakaria MN, Mohamad RA, Nor Rashid MF. Effects of ethnicity and gender on the middle ear function in Asian adults. Indian J Otol 2017;23(2):94-7.

[11] Hall JW. New handbook of auditory evoked responses. Boston, MA: Pearson, 2007.

[12] Abdul Wahab NA, Wahab S, Abdul Rahman AH, Sidek D, Zakaria MN. The hyperactivity of efferent auditory system in patients with schizophrenia: a transient evoked otoacoustic emissions study. Psychiatry Investig 2016;13(1):82-8.

[13] Zakaria MN, Jalaei B, Wahab NA. Gender and modulation frequency effects on auditory steady state response (ASSR) thresholds. Eur Arch Otorhinolaryngol 2016;273(2):349-54.

[14] Jalaei B, Azmi MHAM, Zakaria MN. Gender differences in binaural speech-evoked auditory brainstem response: are they clinically significant? Braz J Otorhinolaryngol 2019;85(4):486-93.

[15] Mukari SZS, Umat C, Chan SC, Ali A, Maamor N, Zakaria MN. Effects of age and type of stimulus on the cortical auditory evoked potential in healthy Malaysian children. J Audiol Otol 2020;24(1):35-9.

[16] Katz J, Marshall C, English K, Hood L, Tillery KL. Handbook of clinical audiology. Philadelphia, PA: Lippincott Williams Wilkins, 2015.

[17] Awang MA, Salim R, Rashid MFN, Mohamad WNW, Omar M, Zakaria MN. The clinical usefulness of the traditional auropalpebral reflex test when assessing a mentally challenged hearing-impaired adult. Otorhinolaryngol Clin 2023;15(1): 48-50.

[18] Zakaria MN, Nik Othman NA, Musa Z. Does the location of electrode on tympanic membrane matter when recording electrocochleography? Acta Otolaryngol 2021;141(11):984-8.

[19] Jalaei B, Zakaria MN, Sidek D. Abnormal auditory brainstem response (ABR) findings in a near-normal hearing child with Noonan syndrome. Iran J Otorhinolaryngol 2017;29(90):53-7.

[20] Rashid MFN, Zakaria MN, Romli M, Mohamad WNW, Awang MA. The presence of atypical auditory brainstem response waveforms in a child with normal hearing. Indian J Otol 2022;28(2):167-70.

[21] Zakaria MN, Jalaei B, Sidek D. Ipsilateral and contralateral recordings of the 40-Hz auditory steady state response (ASSR): Which one is better? B-ENT 2016;12(1):53-7.

[22] Jalaei B, Shaabani M, Zakaria MN. Mode of recording and modulation frequency effects of auditory steady state response thresholds. Braz J Otorhinolaryngol 2017;83(1):10-5.

[23] Cohen LT, Rickards FW, Clark GM. A comparison of steady-state evoked potentials to modulated tones in awake and sleeping humans. J Acoust Soc Am 1991;90(5):2467-79.

[24] Kuwada S, Anderson JS, Batra R, Fitzpatrick DC, Teissier N, D'Angelo WR. Sources of the scalp-recorded amplitude-modulation following response. J Am Acad Audiol 2002;13(4):188-204.

[25] Rance G, Dowell RC, Rickards FW, Beer DE, Clark GM. Steady-state evoked potential and behavioral hearing thresholds in a group of children with absent click-evoked auditory brain stem response. Ear Hear 1998;19(1):48-61.

[26] John MS, Dimitrijevic A, Picton TW. Efficient stimuli for evoking auditory steady-state responses. Ear Hear 2003;24(5):406-23.

[27] Sininger YS, Hunter LL, Hayes D, Roush PA, Uhler KM. Evaluation of speed and accuracy of next-generation auditory steady state response and auditory brainstem response audiometry in children with normal hearing and hearing loss. Ear Hear 2018;39(6):1207-23.

[28] Pethe J, Mühler R, Siewert K, von Specht H. Near-threshold recordings of amplitude modulation following responses (AMFR) in children of different ages. Int J Audiol 2004;43(6):339-45.

[29] Aimoni C, Crema L, Savini S, Negossi L, Rosignoli M, Sacchetto L, et al. Hearing threshold estimation by auditory steady state responses (ASSR) in children. Acta Otorhinolaryngol Ital 2018;38(4):361-8.

[30] Tarawneh HY, Sohrabi HR, Mulders WHAM, Martins RN, Jayakody DMP. Comparison of auditory steady-state responses with conventional audiometry in older adults. Front Neurol 2022;13:924096.

[31] Aslam MA, Javed A, Moiz A. Comparison of auditory brainstem response and auditory steady state response audiometry by evaluating the hearing thresholds obtained in children with different severity of hearing loss. Pak J Med Sci 2019;35(2):320-4.

[32] Korczak P, Smart J, Delgado R, Strobel TM, Bradford C. Auditory steady-state responses. J Am Acad Audiol 2012;23(3):146-70.

[33] Rance G, Rickards FW, Cohen LT, De Vidi S, Clark GM. The automated prediction of hearing thresholds in sleeping subjects using auditory steady-state evoked potentials. Ear Hear 1995;16(5):499-507.

[34] Hosseinabadi R, Jafarzadeh S. Auditory steady-state response thresholds in adults with conductive and mild to moderate sensorineural hearing loss. Iran Red Crescent Med 2014;17(1):e18029.

[35] Vander Werff KR, Brown CJ. Effect of audiometric configuration on threshold and suprathreshold auditory steady-state responses. Ear Hear 2005;26(3):310-26.

[36] Picton TW, Dimitrijevic A, Perez-Abalo MC, Van Roon P. Estimating audiometric thresholds using auditory steady-state responses. J Am Acad Audiol 2005;16(3):140-56.

[37] Chen M, Wei Y, Wang X, Liu L, Liu M, Jiang G, et al. Assessing agreement between frequency-specific chirp auditory steady-state response and pure tone audiometry in adults by intraclass correlation coefficient. ORL J Otorhinolaryngol Relat Spec 2022;84(1):30-8.

[38] Herdman AT, Stapells DK. Auditory steady-state response thresholds of adults with sensorineural hearing impairments. Int J Audiol 2003;42(5):237-48.

[39] DeJonckere PH, Lebacq J. The comparison of auditory behavioral and evoked potential responses (steady state and cortical) in subjects with occupational noise-induced hearing loss. J Otol 2021;16(4):242-51.

[40] van der Reijden CS, Mens LH, Snik AF. Frequency-specific objective audiometry: tone-evoked brainstem responses and steady-state responses to 40 Hz and 90 Hz amplitude modulated stimuli. Int J Audiol 2006;45(1):40-5.

[41] Elberling C, Don M, Cebulla M, Stürzebecher E. Auditory steady-state responses to chirp stimuli based on cochlear traveling wave delay. J Acoust Soc Am 2007;122(5):2772-85.

[42] Zakaria MN, Zainun Z, Cheu Lih A. Considerations when analyzing vestibular evoked myogenic potential (VEMP) outcomes elicited by chirp stimulus in healthy participants. J Int Adv Otol 2015;11(3):271-2.

[43] Lee MY, Ahn SY, Lee HJ, Jung JY, Rhee CK, Suh MW. Narrow band CE-Chirp auditory steady-state response is more reliable than the conventional ASSR in predicting the behavioral hearing threshold. Auris Nasus Larynx 2016;43(3):259-68.

[44] Liu X, Liu S, Guo D, Sheng Y, Ke Y, An X, et al. Enhanced auditory steady-state response using an optimized chirp stimulus-evoked paradigm. Sensors (Basel) 2019;19(3):748.

[45] Wimalarathna H, Ankmnal-Veeranna S, Allan C, Agrawal SK, Samarabandu J, Ladak HM, et al. Machine learning approaches used to analyze auditory evoked responses from the human auditory brainstem: A systematic review. Comput Methods Programs Biomed 2022;226:107118.

[46] Goodfellow I, Bengio Y, Courville A. Deep Learning. Cambridge, MA: MIT Press, 2016.

[47] Buch VH, Ahmed I, Maruthappu M. Artificial intelligence in medicine: current trends and future possibilities. Br J Gen Pract 2018;68(668):143-4.

[48] Chin-Yee B, Upshur R. The impact of artificial intelligence on clinical judgment: a briefing document. Toronto, ON: AMS Healthcare, 2019.

[49] Nayan NA, Jie Yi C, Suboh MZ, Mazlan NF, Periyasamy P, Abdul Rahim MYZ, et al. COVID-19 prediction with machine learning technique from extracted features of photoplethysmogram morphology. Front Public Health 2022;10:920849.

Chapter 4

Aided cortical auditory evoked potential (CAEP) outcomes in hearing-impaired children

Nurnazeha Isnan[1], BSc
Rosninda Abdullah[1], MSc
Mohd FN Rashid[1], PhD
Nik AN Othman[2], MMed
Wan NW Mohamad[1], PhD
Nashrah Maamor[3], PhD
and Mohd N Zakaria[1], PhD

[1]Audiology Programme, School of Health Sciences, Universiti Sains Malaysia, Kelantan, Malaysia
[2]Department of Otorhinolaryngology, School of Medical Sciences, Universiti Sains Malaysia, Kelantan, Malaysia
[3] Centre for Ear, Hearing and Speech, Faculty of Health Sciences, Universiti Kebangsaan Malaysia, Kuala Lumpur, Malaysia

Abstract

Hearing-impaired children with sensorineural hearing loss are typically prescribed with hearing aid (HA). To measure the benefits of HA, various subjective and objective assessments can be conducted. Among the measures, cortical auditory evoked potential (CAEP) is useful to provide objective information regarding the cortical function following the use of HA. As such, the aim of this review was to provide information on the benefits of using HA in light of CAEP studies. Keyword searches using Scopus, PubMed and Google Scholar databases were carried out. In the end, quantitative studies on CAEP in aided hearing-impaired children (n

In: Public Health: Audiology Research in Malaysia
Editors: Mohd N. Zakaria and Joav Merrick
ISBN: 979-8-89530-577-5

= 22) were found to be eligible for review. Analysis of the findings of studies revealed three components that would influence the CAEP outcomes in hearing-impaired children including HA setting, experience factor and language performance. Collectively, we found that there were limited aided CAEP studies in children, in which further research is warranted. Moreover, standardized CAEP normative data are currently lacking, and this aspect should be addressed accordingly in order to develop a suitable protocol to record aided CAEP among children.

Introduction

In both adults and children, hearing impairment and associated auditory disorders are reasonably common (1-6). In children, the number of those with hearing loss is increasing globally. The increase is proportional to high levels of awareness, which leads to higher detection rates in the newborn hearing screening programs. These hearing screening programs are beneficial to detect children with hearing impairment as soon as possible, and late detection of hearing impairment would seriously affect the language, cognitive, and psychosocial development (1, 7).

To accurately diagnose the severity of hearing loss and the type of hearing loss, comprehensive hearing assessments (that consist of objective and subjective tests) are carried out (1, 8, 9). Based on the hearing test results, specific treatment options are then suggested. For children who are diagnosed with sensorineural hearing loss (SNHL), hearing aid (HA) is commonly prescribed (1). The use of HA is important from an early age to ensure the optimal development of auditory skills. There are numerous ways to evaluate the performance of HA, both subjectively and objectively (1,10). Among the assessments, cortical auditory evoked potential (CAEP) is an emerging tool for evaluating the function of HA in hearing-impaired children objectively (10-13).

The CAEP waveforms are produced in response to stimuli such as speech sounds, tone bursts, and others (10, 13). The respective action potentials are generated concurrently within the auditory system and recorded using an auditory evoked potential (AEP) device (and by placing scalp electrodes on specific locations around the head). It consists of prominent peaks including P_1, N_1, P_2, and N_2 with specific amplitudes and latencies (1, 10). As it reflects the function of cortical areas within the auditory system, this electrophysiological test has been studied extensively in normal subjects and those with compromised cortical functions (1, 10, 14, 15).

Studying the influence of hearing amplification devices on the central auditory system may improve scientific understanding of the benefit of auditory rehabilitation (11). To achieve this goal, one viable option is to perform CAEP (due to its objective nature and the fact that it represents the summed neural activity of the auditory cortex in response to sounds). The aided CAEP can be useful for measuring HA outcomes in children, as research on aided CAEP measurement has increased dramatically since 2012. In line with this, Ching et al. (12) reported on the validity of the CAEP method for testing users of HA. As such, the aim of this review was to highlight the CAEP outcomes among HA users (specifically in children).

Our review

The review's principal goal was to determine the impact of children's factors on CAEP findings. Articles (from 2012 to 2021) to be included in the review were mainly identified using SCOPUS, PubMed, and Google Scholar databases using specific keyword searches. The main keywords used were "cortical auditory evoked potential", "hearing aid", "child" and "hearing-impaired" in combination with related synonyms for every keyword that yielded the most relevant materials (see Table 1). The potential articles were also searched using other websites.

The search strategies consisted of identification, screening, and eligibility check to obtain the most relevant articles. The PRISMA checklist (2020) was used to achieve this purpose. Studies to be included must report data on CAEP findings in hearing-impaired children either with or without HA. Case reports, case series and review articles were excluded from this review.

What we found

Figure 1 shows the article search results during the identification and screening stages (using the main databases and other methods). In the end, 22 eligible studies (19 from the main databases and 3 from other websites) were shortlisted and included in the review.

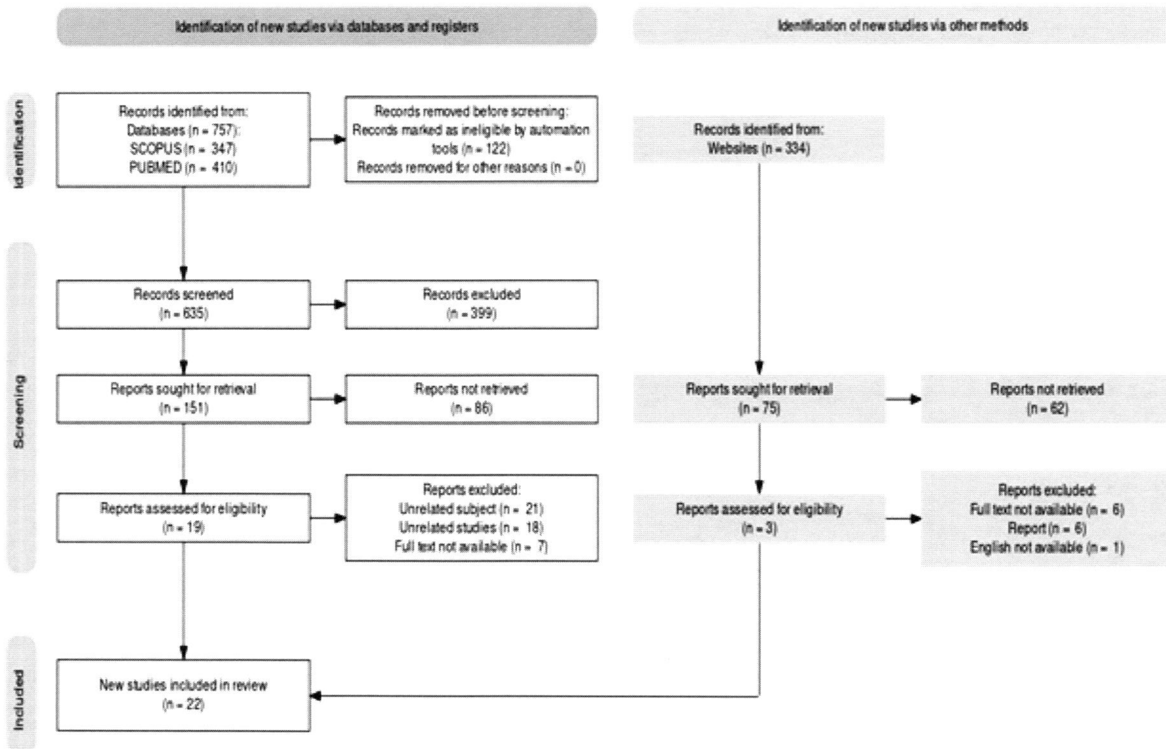

Figure 1. The flow diagram of searching the relevant articles to be included in the review (adapted from PRISMA 2020).

Table 1. Databases and keywords used in the review

Sources	Search String
Scopus	(“cortical auditory evoked potential” OR “auditory evoked potential” OR “auditory late response”) AND (“child” or “pediatric” OR “paediatric”) AND (“hearing aid” OR “hearing instrument” OR “listening device”) AND (“hearing-impaired” OR “hearing impaired” OR “hearing impairment” OR "hearing loss”)
PubMed	((cortical auditory evoked potential) OR (auditory evoked potential) OR (auditory late response)) AND ((child) OR (children) OR (pediatric) OR (paediatric)) AND ((hearing aid) OR (hearing instrument) OR (listening device)) AND ((hearing-impaired) OR (hearing impaired) OR (hearing impairment) OR (hearing loss))
Google Scholar	(“cortical” OR “auditory evoked response” OR “auditory late response”) AND (“hearing aid” OR “hearing instrument” OR “listening device”) AND (child OR children OR pediatric OR paediatric) AND (“hearing-impaired” OR “hearing loss”)

Discussion

The key articles included provide information on the methods used to measure the CAEP benefits through comparisons. This review found three methods: first, comparing the hearing-impaired group to the reference group (normal hearing), second, comparing the pre-rehabilitation with post-rehabilitation CAEP within a specific period (pre- and post-study), and third, comparing the unaided to aided CAEP in hearing-impaired subjects (with and without HA).

The first method for comparing CAEP findings between groups was to document the benefits of HA in hearing-impaired children who would exhibit improved CAEP waveforms after the intervention. Most of the key articles in this review employed this method to assess the benefits and outcomes of HA. The second method was a pre- and post-study assessing the benefits of HA using CAEP before and after the intervention. Herein, the application of CAEP has both advantages and disadvantages in the pre- and post-study design. This study design is relatively convenient as it can be used in any studies that measure the effect of HA technology on individual subjects (by means of CAEP). The disadvantage of using this method is that the dropout rate can be high because the subjects must attend the experiment twice. On the other hand, the third method compared the unaided and aided CAEP outcomes to observe the changes that would reflect the benefits of HA.

Based on the review results, the subject effect of hearing impairment can be explained by three CAEP indicators including HA setting, experience factor and language performance. These factors are described accordingly in this review.

HA setting

In hearing-impaired children who use HA, a variety of prescriptions need to be verified and validated. Korczak et al. (16) discovered a method for evaluating the effectiveness of HA in adults using the aided CAEP in earlier years. Since reliable speech perception results are frequently impossible to obtain among young children, the application of CAEP can be useful in this situation. In line with this, studies on CAEP demonstrated that this electrophysiological test can be an objective tool for measuring the benefits of frequency compression (FC) or HA fitting formula/rule (12, 17). The amplified stimulus effect (due to the HA use) would influence the CAEP waveforms, as well as the type of stimulus to evoke CAEP. Owing to this, CAEP amplitudes and latencies may provide concrete evidence that different spectral levels of speech sounds are encoded differently at the cortical regions (18).

Divergent conclusions about CAEP amplitudes, latencies, and morphology can be drawn from the perspective of HA technology or the HA formula. Some HA employs the frequency compression technique to enhance the audibility of high-frequency sounds. By making the 4 kHz tone burst more audible through the use of frequency compression technology, CAEP responses could be identified more accurately. This outcome suggests that the CAEP is vulnerable to the effects of frequency compression signal processing and that, depending on the circumstances, frequency compression may have made high-frequency tone bursts more audible (19). In line with this, Ching et al. (12) found that the frequency compression technique would enhance the CAEP detection rate in children at the conversational level. Additionally, Golding et al. (20) discovered that the existence of CAEP waves indicated that the HA gave young infants adequate gain at the conversational level in response to speech sounds. A different approach to gain understanding on the benefits of HA was to consider the sensation levels used to evoke CAEP. In this regard, the relationship between CAEP and sensation level would vary between hearing-impaired and normal hearing children, resulting in higher sensation levels in the hearing-impaired group and greater amplitudes in the aided CAEP compared to normal hearing children.

Experience with HA use

The CAEP results may provide an explanation of the experience with HA. The accumulated evidence suggests that P1 is a reliable peak when assessing users' experiences with HA. For instance, after using appropriate HA for 15 months, CAEP results typically improve to normal values in children (21). Furthermore, in a study conducted by Leite et al. (22), the P1 peak was used as a biomarker to document changes in the cortical auditory pathway after the use of HA or cochlear implant. They discovered that the P1 peak dominated the CAEP, appearing in 100% of normal children. On the other hand, the P1 peak was longer in latency in the hearing-impaired users, reflecting the inconsistent use of HA.

The CAEP results for children wearing HA demonstrated a progressive correlation with parental questionnaires (20). This suggests that wearing HA can enhance audibility, which will increase the capacity to identify CAEP responses. Furthermore, at the suprathreshold stimulus levels, it provides electrophysiological evidence that the stimuli are in fact detected in the auditory cortex with the use of HA (19). In contrast, it is delayed by the duration of deafness due to its effect on the auditory plasticity (23). In accordance with this, as shown by CAEP results, lack of audibility experienced by children with SNHL would result in significant deficits and delays in the auditory cortical maturation (24). That is, less experience would lead to significant reductions or interruptions to the auditory cortex in children, as well as the development of brain plasticity.

Language performance

Language development will be hampered by hearing impairment. In this regard, hearing-impaired children who did not have language impairment may exhibit normal CAEP responses. In contrast, children with language impairment would show abnormal CAEP results including the absence of CAEP peaks. Furthermore, Bakhos et al. (25) found that the language ability would predict the auditory inputs provided by the HA. Additionally, this study recommended the temporal scalp recording of CAEP, as it was found to represent the secondary auditory cortex (that underlies language impairment), particularly in children with moderate SNHL (25). Consistent with other reports, hearing impairment would impede the normal development of the connectivity necessary for the formation of a functional auditory system that contributes to language development.

Conclusion

The aided CAEP assessment is able to provide objective information regarding the function of the auditory cortex in hearing-impaired children. This is particularly useful when assessing the HA benefits involving "difficult-to-test" children and complex paediatric cases. Based on the review outcomes, the number of studies emphasizing the application of CAEP in children with HA was inadequate. This could be due to many potential factors that should be addressed accordingly. Given the fact that children's auditory maturation and development are still ongoing, there are still no available standards and norms for recording CAEP, even among normal hearing children. Although more research efforts are needed, evaluating the aided CAEP (elicited by different speech stimuli) in hearing-impaired children may potentially provide important insights into the higher-order brain functions (resulting from the continuous use of HA). By combining data from many studies, a standardized and effective protocol for documenting CAEP in children can be developed.

References

[1] Katz J, Marshall C, English K, Hood L, Tillery KL. Handbook of clinical audiology. Philadelphia: Lippincott Williams Wilkins, 2015.

[2] Wan Mohamad WN, Romli M, Awang MA, Abdullah R, Lih AC, Zakaria MN. The presence of unusual bone conduction thresholds in pure tone audiometry. Indian J Otol 2020;26(1):54-7.

[3] Wong JW, Wan Mohamad WN, Wan Husain WS, Zakaria MN. The tinnitus suppressive effect: Comparisons between three types of maskers. Int J Disabil Hum Dev 2020;19(1):21-6.

[4] Zakaria MN. The effectiveness of sound therapy in treating patients with mild and severe tinnitus. Int J Disabil Hum Dev 2020;19(2):215-9.

[5] Wahab S, Zakaria MN, Sidek D, Abdul Rahman AH, Shah SA, Abdul Wahab NA. Evaluation of auditory hallucinations in patients with schizophrenia: A validation study of the Malay version of Psychotic Symptom Rating Scales (PSYRATS). Psychiatry Res 2015;228(3):462-7.

[6] Abdul Wahab NA, Wahab S, Abdul Rahman AH, Sidek D, Zakaria MN. The hyperactivity of efferent auditory system in patients with schizophrenia: a transient evoked otoacoustic emissions study. Psychiatr Investig 2016;13(1):82-8.

[7] Vos B, Noll D, Pigeon M, Bagatto M, Fitzpatrick EM. Risk factors for hearing loss in children: a systematic literature review and meta-analysis protocol. Syst Rev 2019;8(1):172.

[8] Romli M, Wan Mohamad WN, Awang MA, Aw CL, Zakaria MN. The clinical value of bilateral bone conduction testing in hearing diagnosis. Indian J Otol 2020;26(3):182-5.

[9] Lih AC, Zakaria MN, Mohamad RA, Nor Rashid MF. Effects of ethnicity and gender on the middle ear function in Asian adults. Indian J Otol 2017;23(2):94-7.

[10] Hall JW. New handbook of auditory evoked responses. Boston, MA: Pearson, 2007.

[11] Billings CJ, Tremblay KL, Souza PE, Binns MA. Effects of hearing aid amplification and stimulus intensity on cortical auditory evoked potentials. Audiol Neurootol 2007;12(4):234-46.

[12] Ching TY, Zhang VW, Hou S, Van Buynder P. Cortical auditory evoked potentials reveal changes in audibility with nonlinear frequency compression in hearing aids for children: clinical implications. Semin Hear 2016;37(1):25-35.

[13] Mukari SZS, Umat C, Chan SC, Ali A, Maamor N, Zakaria MN. Effects of age and type of stimulus on the cortical auditory evoked potential in healthy Malaysian children. J Audiol Otol 2020;24(1):35-9.

[14] Sharma A, Cardon G. Cortical development and neuroplasticity in Auditory Neuropathy Spectrum Disorder. Hear Res 2015;330(Pt B):221-32.

[15] Távora-Vieira D, Wedekind A, Ffoulkes E, Voola M, Marino R. Cortical auditory evoked potential in cochlear implant users: An objective method to improve speech perception. PLoS One 2022;17(10):e0274643.

[16] Korczak PA, Kurtzberg D, Stapells DR. Effects of sensorineural hearing loss and personal hearing AIDS on cortical event-related potential and behavioral measures of speech-sound processing. Ear Hear 2005;26(2):165-85.

[17] Hazzaa N, Hassan DM, Hassan A. Evaluation of non-linear frequency compression hearing aids using speech P1-cortical auditory evoked potential. Hear Balance Commun 2016;14(1):36-43.

[18] Almeqbel A. Speech-evoked cortical auditory responses in children with normal hearing. S Afr J Commun Disord 2013;60:38-43.

[19] Glista D, Easwar V, Purcell DW, Scollie S. A pilot study on cortical auditory evoked potentials in children: aided CAEPs reflect improved high-frequency audibility with frequency compression hearing aid technology. Int J Otolaryngol 2012;2012:982894.

[20] Golding M, Pearce W, Seymour J, Cooper A, Ching T, Dillon H. The relationship between obligatory cortical auditory evoked potentials (CAEPs) and functional measures in young infants. J Am Acad Audiol 2007;18(2):117-25.

[21] El-Sharnouby MK, El-Mousely MM, Ragab AA, El-Abedein AM. Validity of P1 testing as an objective tool for hearing aid verification in children. Menoufia Med J 2015;28:213-8.

[22] Leite RA, Magliaro FCL, Raimundo JC, Bento RF, Matas CG. Monitoring auditory cortical plasticity in hearing aid users with long latency auditory evoked potentials: a longitudinal study. Clinics (Sao Paulo) 2018;73:e51.

[23] Koravand A, Jutras B, Lassonde M. Cortical auditory evoked potentials in children with a hearing loss: a pilot study. Int J Pediatr 2012;2012:250254.
[24] Sharma A, Martin K, Roland P, Bauer P, Sweeney MH, Gilley P, et al. P1 latency as a biomarker for central auditory development in children with hearing impairment. J Am Acad Audiol 2005;16(8):564-73.
[25] Bakhos D, Delage H, Galvin J, Lescanne E, Roux S, Bonnet-Brilhault F, et al. Cortical electrophysiological markers of language abilities in children with hearing AIDS: A pilot study. Biomed Res Int 2014;2014:198153.

Chapter 5

Understanding the neural processing of cochlear implant users: Insights from cortical auditory evoked potential (CAEP) findings

Rosninda Abdullah[1], MSc
Noor AA Wahab[1], PhD
Nashrah Maamor[2], PhD
Nik AN Othman[3], MMed
Basyariatul F Othman[2], PhD
and Mohd N Zakaria[4], PhD

[1]Audiology Programme, Centre for Rehabilitation and Special Needs Studies, Faculty of Health Sciences, Universiti Kebangsaan Malaysia, Kuala Lumpur, Malaysia
[2]Centre for Ear, Hearing and Speech, Faculty of Health Sciences, Universiti Kebangsaan Malaysia, Kuala Lumpur, Malaysia
[3]Department of Otorhinolaryngology, School of Medical Sciences, Universiti Sains Malaysia, Kelantan, Malaysia, and [4]Audiology Programme, School of Health Sciences, Universiti Sains Malaysia, Kelantan, Malaysia

Abstract

Cochlear implants (CIs) are electronic devices fitted on individuals with severe and profound deafness that are effective in improving hearing and speech perception. In children, obtaining the optimum map setting of CIs is important, and this can be achieved using subjective or objective measures. The cortical auditory evoked potential (CAEP) has been gaining interest among researchers and clinicians as it is able to assess the outcomes of CIs among paediatric population in an objective manner. In this chapter, the importance of having CIs and appropriate CI mapping

In: Public Health: Audiology Research in Malaysia
Editors: Mohd N. Zakaria and Joav Merrick
ISBN: 979-8-89530-577-5

is highlighted as intended. Fundamental information about CAEP and factors affecting its results are reviewed accordingly. The potential use of this objective assessment in measuring the benefits of CIs is emphasized. According to the available research findings, more CAEP studies are required to fully investigate and apprehend the usefulness of this objective measure in children with CIs. Among other things, comparing the performance of electrical and acoustic CAEP can provide useful information regarding which stimulation is better for measuring CI outcomes.

Introduction

Depending on the type and severity of hearing loss, hearing-impaired children and adults require specific treatments and/or intervention strategies (1-3). Those who are diagnosed with conductive hearing loss (CHL) are typically treated medically and/or surgically. Meanwhile, due to permanent damage to the inner ear, the use of hearing amplification devices is recommended for hearing-impaired individuals diagnosed with sensorineural hearing loss (SNHL). In particular, patients with mild to severe SNHL are fitted with hearing aids (1), while cochlear implants (CIs) are chosen for profound hearing loss cases (3, 4).

The CI is a complex electronic device that can help individuals (who are profoundly deaf) to understand speech and develop spoken language skills (4). Generally, it works by converting sounds into electrical signals. Herein, it bypasses the damaged parts of the inner ear and directly stimulates the auditory nerve. These signals are then sent to the brainstem and brain. The brain interprets these signals as sounds. The CI device consists of two main parts: the external part, which is worn behind the ear and includes a microphone and a speech processor, and the internal part, which is surgically implanted under the skin behind the ear. The internal part includes an electrode array that sends electrical signals to the auditory nerve. The implantation process involves surgery that is usually conducted on an outpatient basis. After the surgery, the CI device will be switched on, and mapping procedures will be carried out (3). The patient will also need to undergo a period of rehabilitation and training to learn how to use the implant effectively. In line with advancements in technology (and how it has evolved over the years), this hearing implant is able to provide improved sound quality and have been shown to be effective in both adults and children (5, 6).

The mapping of CI is a crucial step in the process of optimizing the device's performance for CI recipients (1,3). In this procedure, the audiologist will adjust the settings of the CI device to ensure that it is delivering appropriate levels of electrical stimulation to different parts of the cochlea. This process involves measuring the individual's perception of sounds and making fine-tuned adjustments to maximize speech understanding and overall hearing quality. Ultimately, the threshold (T) level and most comfortable level (MCL) are measured for every implanted electrode. By customizing the CI settings through mapping, the CI recipients can experience improved speech understanding and overall hearing quality tailored to their individual needs and preferences. Both subjective and objective assessments can be used for CI mapping. Nevertheless, CI mapping with subjective measures can be challenging, particularly when dealing with young children (7). Having objective measurements for CI mapping is beneficial in light of this. Electrically evoked stapedial reflex threshold (ESRT), electrical compound action potential (eCAP), and electrical auditory brainstem response (eABR) are among the common objective assessments for CI mapping (3, 8, 9).

Cortical auditory evoked potential (CAEP)

Auditory evoked potentials (AEPs) have many applications in clinical practice (10). They represent electrical responses in the auditory pathway that occur in response to auditory stimulations. By having electrodes placed on specific areas of the head, the sum of time-locked electrical potentials is obtained, and the respective waveforms are displayed for interpretation. This objective assessment provides valuable insights into the neural processing of auditory stimuli and can be used to study various aspects of auditory perception, including sound processing and language processing, in healthy and pathological subjects (10). Electrocochleography (ECochG), auditory brainstem response (ABR), auditory middle latency response (AMLR), auditory steady state response (ASSR), and auditory late response (ALR) are AEPs that have been used commonly for specific clinical purposes (10-15).

The ALR can be used to document neurophysiological changes that occur in the cortical regions of the auditory pathway concerning specific skills that include attention, auditory discrimination, integration, and memory (16). The cortical auditory evoked potential (CAEP) is a type of ALR that has piqued interest among many researchers (10). The neural responses of CAEP are believed to originate from areas that include the primary auditory cortex and the thalamic and auditory association areas (1, 10). It can be evoked by various types of stimuli including clicks, tones, and speech sounds across the life span, of infants (17, 18), young children (19, 20), adolescents (21, 22), young adults (22-24), and the elderly (25). The P1, N1, and P2 components of CAEP are obligatory responses, which are typically recorded using a passive listening paradigm, with the listener watching a silent subtitled video or reading. Infants can be tested while they are awake and distracted by a visually engaging toy or book or during ''active'' sleep (17).

There are several factors that can affect CAEP results. Most notably, the prominent peaks of CAEP are affected by maturation (19-22). For example, the mean P1 latency in neonates with normal hearing is approximately 300 ms. There is a sharp decline in latency during the first two to three years of life (to about 125 ms at age three), followed by a more gradual decline into the second decade. In adults with normal hearing (ages 22-25), the mean P1 latency is around 60 ms (26). The neural travel time in response to auditory stimulation is indicated by these latency values, with P1 latency, in particular, reflecting the total sum of synaptic propagation delays through the central and peripheral auditory pathways (27).

The CAEP waveforms are also influenced by the type of stimulus used in the CAEP testing. Tones and speech sounds are the typical stimuli employed to record CAEP waveforms (1, 10, 15). The tone-evoked CAEP can be conveniently recorded using the standard two-channel AEP machine available in many clinics. The tones used are the standard frequency-specific tone bursts, which can be tested at a single frequency (such as at 500 Hz, 1 kHz, 2 kHz, or 4 kHz). On the other hand, speech stimuli may consist of syllables or phonemes, which are more natural and contain multiple frequencies (10). In view of this, different stimuli may produce different CAEP findings. Mukari et al. (15) compared CAEP latencies between tone-evoked CAEP and speech-evoked CAEP among Malay children with normal-hearing sensitivity aged between 4 and 12 years. They then found a negative significant correlation between the speech-evoked CAEP latency and the age of children. In contrast, for the tone-evoked CAEP, there was no significant correlation between the latency and amplitude of CAEP and the children's age. Additionally, this study also revealed that the speech syllable /ba/ produced a higher mean P1 amplitude compared to the tonal stimulus. In line with this, a study by Ibrahim et al. (28) also found a larger P1 amplitude for the speech-evoked CAEP relative to the tone burst. Collectively, to elicit more robust CAEP waveforms, complex stimuli (such as speech sounds) should be prioritized.

CAEP findings in CI users

The CAEP procedure can be used for various applications, including assessing the maturation of the auditory system, auditory processing ability, and speech audibility in infants and children with hearing loss (24, 29, 30). Additionally, this objective measure can be used to assist in device programming and CI mapping (31), estimate an individual's suprathreshold processing abilities (32), and examine plasticity-related changes that occur in the brain during auditory rehabilitation or intervention sessions (33, 34).

There are at least two ways to obtain CAEP results from targeted patients or subjects who are fitted with CIs. First, by using acoustic stimuli such as tones or speech tokens, which are presented via a loudspeaker, i.e., the acoustic CAEP (aCAEP) method. When measuring CAEP waveforms, a child is seated in a calibrated position, and the stimuli are presented at a suprathreshold level (which is usually at the child's comfortable intensity level) (Figure 1). The CAEP waveforms are then recorded and interpreted accordingly. Second, the CAEP responses can be obtained by delivering electrical stimulation, i.e., the electrical CAEP (eCAEP) method. In this procedure, the electrical current is triggered by the dedicated CI programming software, bypasses the speech processor, and is directly transmitted to the auditory nerve through selected electrodes of the CI device (Figure 2). The CI software is connected to the AEP device through a "trigger-in" cable, and CAEP waveforms (resulting from the electrical stimulation) are produced for interpretation.

In some studies, the HEARLab® system (Frye Electronics, Oregon, USA) was used for the speech-evoked aCAEP recording (31, 35, 36). Employing specific speech phonemes, this AEP system is suitable for assessing normal-hearing subjects or those who are fitted with hearing aids or CIs. The speech tokens, having different characteristic frequencies, can be played at predetermined stimulation levels to elicit aCAEP waveforms to objectively evaluate the auditory cortical regions at different frequency ranges and are therefore potentially useful to guide the establishment of MCL among CI users in clinical settings.

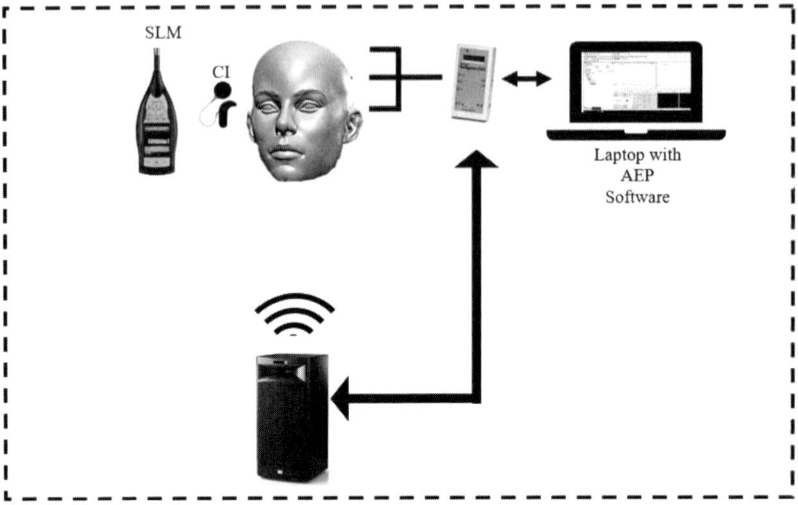

Figure 1. The test setup of the acoustic cortical auditory evoked potential (aCAEP) procedure.

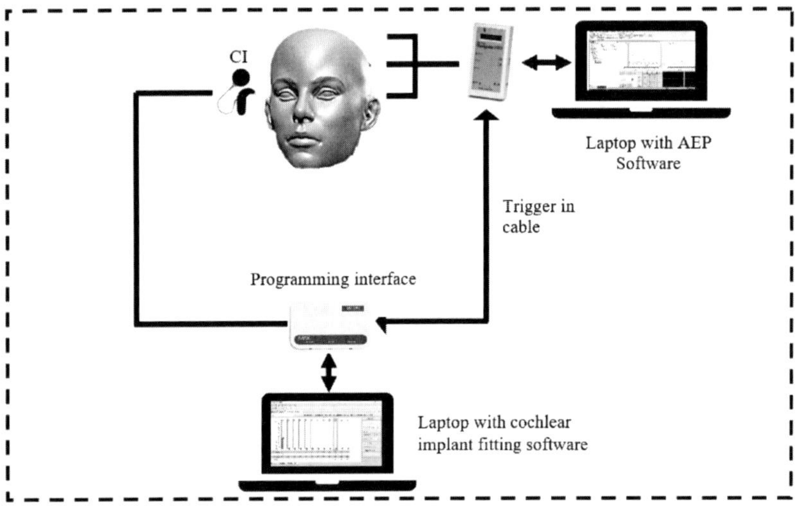

Figure 2. The test setup of the electrical cortical auditory evoked potential (eCAEP) procedure.

In a study involving 44 adult CI users, Liebscher et al. (37) demonstrated that it is possible to generate suitable stimulation patterns for eCAEP from the fitting software of the CI manufacturers, thereby bypassing the audio processor and the conversion from acoustic to electric stimuli. In line with this,

Tavora-Vieira et al. (38) recorded aCAEP and eCAEP responses from 20 adult CI recipients. Specifically, they aimed to compare the amplitude and latency of the P1-N1-P2 complex of eCAEP with those of aCAEP after recording eCAEP at MCL and 50% MCL settings using three CI electrodes (apical, middle, and basal). For obtaining aCAEP waveforms, this study utilized the HEARLab® system, and the stimuli were phonemes (i.e., /m/, /g/, /t/, and /s/). Depending on the type of speech phoneme, aCAEP responses were present in 90%-100% of the subjects. In the eCAEP testing, when the apical and middle electrodes were stimulated, N1 and P2 peaks could be seen, but the P1 peak was less evident for all stimulated electrodes. They also reported that in comparison to MCL, there was an overall increase in latencies for stimulation at 50% MCL. The amplitudes of P1-N1 and N1-P2 were reported to be statistically different between 50% MCL and MCL settings. Based on the eCAEP findings, this study supports the use of appropriate MCL settings in CI mapping to optimize speech perception among CI users.

So far, due to limited literature, it is uncertain regarding the most optimum method to elicit CAEP responses in CI users (i.e., either acoustically or electrically). Apart from the robustness of CAEP waveforms, each method has its own advantages and limitations. The use of various options of speech stimuli is able to provide realistic listening environments, and it is sensible to "directly" compare the resultant aCAEP waveforms with children's auditory and speech abilities. Nevertheless, a soundproof room (with adequate space) and an external loudspeaker (with proper calibration) are needed in this aCAEP testing. On the other hand, the eCAEP method has several benefits (37, 38). First, it can provide more precise and controlled electrical stimulation in terms of level, stimulating electrode, burst length, and burst rate. Second, there is no need for an acoustic-soundproof room with a calibrated setup. Third, focused electrical stimulation can be applied to certain electrodes without being affected by the background electrical stimulation (generated by the audio processor of CI device). Fourth, it does not activate channels that do not represent the frequency of the acoustic stimuli. Finally, it can easily be applied using any AEP device that has the CAEP recording module and the "trigger-in" option. However, compared to the aCAEP method, this procedure is less realistic and may not provide "direct" information regarding speech perception in natural listening environments. Moreover, some electrodes may not produce identifiable CAEP peaks (and it is unknown whether this is due to "poor" auditory skills or technical issues).

Future directions

In line with technological advancements and ongoing research efforts, modern CI devices are able to provide improved sound access, fostering better speech and language development in hearing-impaired children. Among the critical aspects of CIs is ensuring that the mapping is optimal. In view of this, having an objective assessment such as CAEP can be beneficial. Furthermore, it is still unknown as to which stimulation method (acoustic CAEP vs. electrical CAEP) is better at evoking stable CAEP waveforms as well as providing better mapping outcomes (that correlate with auditory and speech skills), particularly in children. Compared to other AEPs (e.g., eCAP or eABR), less research was conducted in regard to eCAEP among children with CIs. As such, further studies on this interesting aspect of CIs are highly encouraged.

References

[1] Katz J, Marshall C, English K, Hood L, Tillery KL. Handbook of clinical audiology. Philadelphia: Lippincott Williams Wilkins, 2015.

[2] Romli M, Wan Mohamad WN, Awang MA, Aw CL, Zakaria MN. The clinical value of bilateral bone conduction testing in hearing diagnosis. Indian J Otol 2020;26(3):182-5.

[3] Aw CL, Tan SK, Abdullah R, Othman NAN, Zakaria MN. Electrically evoked stapedial reflex threshold assessment among Malaysian cochlear implant users: Comparisons between different stimulus rates. Indian J Otol 2020;26(2):89-92.

[4] Hassan MNHC, Mohamad WNW, Awang MA, Maamor N, Wahab NAA, Zakaria MN. Does the auditory localization ability improve with the use of cochlear implant? Int J Disabil Hum Dev 2021;20(3):237-42.

[5] Bond M, Mealing S, Anderson R, Elston J, Weiner G, Taylor RS, et al. The effectiveness and cost-effectiveness of cochlear implants for severe to profound deafness in children and adults: a systematic review and economic model. Health Technol Assess 2009;13(44):1-330.

[6] Sharma SD, Cushing SL, Papsin BC, Gordon KA. Hearing and speech benefits of cochlear implantation in children: A review of the literature. Int J Pediatr Otorhinolaryngol 2020;133:109984.

[7] Langman AW, Quigley SM, Souliere CR Jr. Cochlear implants in children. Pediatr Clin North Am 1996;43:1217-31.

[8] Kosaner J, Spitzer P, Bayguzina S, Gultekin M, Behar LA. Comparing eSRT and eCAP measurements in pediatric MED-EL cochlear implant users. Cochlear Implants Int 2018;19(3):153-161.

[9] Wang Y, Pan T, Deshpande SB, Ma F. The relationship between eABR and auditory performance and speech intelligibility outcomes in pediatric cochlear implant recipients. Am J Audiol 2015;24(2):226-34.

[10] Hall JW. New handbook of auditory evoked responses. Boston, MA: Pearson, 2007.

[11] Zakaria MN, Nik Othman NA, Musa Z. Electrocochleographic recording in Asian adults: Preliminary normative data and demographic analyses. J Otol 2017;12(1):29-33.

[12] Zakaria MN, Wahab NAA, Maamor N, Jalaei B, Dzulkarnain AAA. Auditory brainstem response (ABR) findings in males and females with comparable head sizes at supra-threshold and threshold levels. Neurol Psychiatry Brain Res 2019;32:4-7.

[13] Jalaei B, Azmi MHAM, Zakaria MN. Gender differences in binaural speech-evoked auditory brainstem response: are they clinically significant? Braz J Otorhinolaryngol 2019;85(4):486-93.

[14] Zakaria MN, Jalaei B, Wahab NA. Gender and modulation frequency effects on auditory steady state response (ASSR) thresholds. Eur Arch Otorhinolaryngol 2016;273(2):349-54.

[15] Mukari SZS, Umat C, Chan SC, Ali A, Maamor N, Zakaria MN. Effects of age and type of stimulus on the cortical auditory evoked potential in healthy Malaysian children. J Audiol Otol 2020;24(1):35-9.

[16] Perez AP, Ziliotto K, Pereira LD. Test-retest of long latency auditory evoked potentials (P300) with pure tone and speech stimuli. Int Arch Otorhinolaryngol 2017;21(2):134-9.

[17] Munro KJ, Purdy SC, Uus K, Visram A, Ward R, Bruce IA, et al. Recording obligatory cortical auditory evoked potentials in infants: quantitative information on feasibility and parent acceptability. Ear Hear 2020;41(3):630-9.

[18] Visram AS, Stone MA, Purdy SC, Bell SL, Brooks J, Bruce IA, et al. Aided cortical auditory evoked potentials in infants with frequency-specific synthetic speech stimuli: sensitivity, repeatability, and feasibility. Ear Hear 2023;44(5):1157-72.

[19] Sharma A, Kraus N, McGee TJ, Nicol TG. Developmental changes in P1 and N1 central auditory responses elicited by consonant-vowel syllables. Electroencephalogr Clin Neurophysiol 1997;104(6):540-5.

[20] Ceponiene R, Rinne T, Näätänen R. Maturation of cortical sound processing as indexed by event-related potentials. Clin Neurophysiol 2002;113(6):870-82.

[21] Ponton CW, Don M, Eggermont JJ, Waring MD, Masuda A. Maturation of human cortical auditory function: differences between normal-hearing children and children with cochlear implants. Ear Hear 1996;17(5):430-7.

[22] Cunningham J, Nicol T, Zecker S, Kraus N. Speech-evoked neurophysiologic responses in children with learning problems: development and behavioral correlates of perception. Ear Hear 2000;21(6):554-68.

[23] Wunderlich JL, Cone-Wesson BK. Effects of stimulus frequency and complexity on the mismatch negativity and other components of the cortical auditory-evoked potential. J Acoust Soc Am 2001;109(4):1526-37.

[24] Sharma A, Dorman MF, Spahr AJ. A sensitive period for the development of the central auditory system in children with cochlear implants: implications for age of implantation. Ear Hear 2002;23(6):532-9.

[25] Lister JJ, Harrison Bush AL, Andel R, Matthews C, Morgan D, Edwards JD. Cortical auditory evoked responses of older adults with and without probable mild cognitive impairment. Clin Neurophysiol 2016;127(2):1279-87.

[26] Dorman MF, Sharma A, Gilley P, Martin K, Roland P. Central auditory development: evidence from CAEP measurements in children fit with cochlear implants. J Commun Disord 2007;40(4):284-94.

[27] Eggermont JJ, Ponton CW, Don M, Waring MD, Kwong B. Maturational delays in cortical evoked potentials in cochlear implant users. Acta Otolaryngol 1997;117(2):161-3.

[28] Ibrahim IA, Ting HN, Moghavvemi M. The effects of audio stimuli on auditory-evoked potential in normal hearing Malay adults. Int J Health Sci (Qassim) 2018;12(5):25-34.

[29] Golding M, Pearce W, Seymour J, Cooper A, Ching T, Dillon H. The relationship between obligatory cortical auditory evoked potentials (CAEPs) and functional measures in young infants. J Am Acad Audiol 2007;18(2):117-25.

[30] Martin BA, Tremblay KL, Korczak P. Speech evoked potentials: from the laboratory to the clinic. Ear Hear 2008;29(3):285-313.

[31] Távora-Vieira D, Wedekind A, Marino R, Purdy SC, Rajan GP. Using aided cortical assessment as an objective tool to evaluate cochlear implant fitting in users with single-sided deafness. PLoS One 2018;13(2):e0193081.

[32] Hyde M. The N1 response and its applications. Audiol Neurootol 1997;2(5):281-307.

[33] Alvarenga KF, Amorim RB, Agostinho-Pesse RS, Costa OA, Nascimento LT, Bevilacqua MC. Speech perception and cortical auditory evoked potentials in cochlear implant users with auditory neuropathy spectrum disorders. Int J Pediatr Otorhinolaryngol 2012;76(9):1332-8.

[34] Guo Q, Li Y, Fu X, Liu H, Chen J, Meng C, et al. The relationship between cortical auditory evoked potentials (CAEPs) and speech perception in children with Nurotron® cochlear implants during four years of follow-up. Int J Pediatr Otorhinolaryngol 2016;85:170-7.

[35] Munro KJ, Purdy SC, Ahmed S, Begum R, Dillon H. Obligatory cortical auditory evoked potential waveform detection and differentiation using a commercially available clinical system: HEARLab™. Ear Hear 2011;32(6):782-6.

[36] Mehta K, Watkin P, Baldwin M, Marriage J, Mahon M, Vickers D. Role of cortical auditory evoked potentials in reducing the age at hearing aid fitting in children with hearing loss identified by newborn hearing screening. Trends Hear 2017;21:2331216517744094.

[37] Liebscher T, Alberter K, Hoppe U. Cortical auditory evoked potentials in cochlear implant listeners via single electrode stimulation in relation to speech perception. Int J Audiol 2018;57(12):933-40.

[38] Távora-Vieira D, Mandruzzato G, Polak M, Truong B, Stutley A. Comparative analysis of cortical auditory evoked potential in cochlear implant users. Ear Hear 2021;42(6):1755-69.

Chapter 6

Managing patients with tinnitus: The potential role of teleaudiology

Shameera Nizamuddin[1,2], BSc
Mohd N Zakaria[2], PhD
Mohd FN Rashid[2], PhD
Wan SW Husain[3], MSc
and Wan NW Mohamad[2], PhD
[1]Hospital Cyberjaya, Putrajaya, Wilayah Persekutuan Putrajaya, Malaysia
[2]Audiology Programme, School of Health Sciences, Universiti Sains Malaysia, Kelantan, Malaysia
[3]Hospital Sultanah Nur Zahirah, Jalan Sultan Mahmud, Kuala Terengganu, Malaysia

Abstract

Tinnitus ("ringing sound in the ear") is a prevalent and yet serious symptom among adults with ear problems. Due to its negative impacts on the well-being of the affected individuals, timely assessments and interventions are therefore necessary. In clinical settings, audiologists are the primary clinicians who play a notable role in evaluating and treating those with tinnitus. The implementation of telehealth has introduced a new revolution in the field of medicine with many great advantages. In line with this, there has been a growing interest in studying the usefulness of teleaudiology in service delivery. More recently, the application of teleaudiology in the field of tinnitus has been initiated by several researchers. In this chapter, the impacts of tinnitus on various aspects of life are described accordingly. The use of teleaudiology in specific clinical tasks, as well as its advantages and disadvantages, are highlighted as intended. In addition, factors that determine the success of this

In: Public Health: Audiology Research in Malaysia
Editors: Mohd N. Zakaria and Joav Merrick
ISBN: 979-8-89530-577-5

telehealth service are also discussed. Based on the current literature, more research efforts are needed to promote the application of teleaudiology in assessing and managing patients with tinnitus. It appears crucial to evaluate the acceptance of teleaudiology among both healthcare practitioners and patients (with different demographic backgrounds), and this is subject to future research.

Introduction

In both adults and children, hearing impairment and associated auditory disorders are reasonably common (1-7). Tinnitus, i.e., the perception of sounds in the ear or head, is a serious symptom that requires specialised assessments and rehabilitation techniques (8, 9). Frequently, the sounds perceived are described as ringing, hissing, buzzing, or clicking. The affected individuals may experience intermittent (pulsatile type) or continuous tinnitus (8).

Tinnitus can be caused by different factors, including exposure to loud noises, age-related hearing loss, earwax blockage, certain medications, and underlying health conditions (10). It is often a symptom of an underlying issue rather than a standalone condition. Since the common cause of tinnitus is the cochlear damage (8, 10), and it rarely "disappears", most of the patients must "live" with their tinnitus throughout their lives. Even though more options are now available for treating tinnitus (i.e., psychoeducation, hearing aids, sound therapy, cognitive behavioural therapy, etc.) (11-14), ongoing efforts are needed to search for the best treatments for tinnitus, and continuous consultations and counselling sessions are useful to assist patients in dealing with their tinnitus problems.

Tinnitus and its impacts

The effects of tinnitus can vary greatly from person to person (15). For some individuals, tinnitus may be a minor annoyance that does not significantly impact their daily life. However, for others, it can be extremely disruptive and have negative impacts on their quality of life (8-10). The impacts of tinnitus can be seen in various aspects such as difficulties with attention and concentration, sleep disturbances, and can potentially result in psychological distress.

The persistent ringing or buzzing sounds can make it challenging for patients with tinnitus to concentrate on tasks, especially those that require focus or attention (16). Daily activities such as work, studying, or conversations may become more difficult. Tinnitus can also interfere with sleep patterns, making it difficult to fall asleep or stay asleep. Lack of quality sleep can further contribute to emotional distress and overall fatigue (17).

The emergence of psychological problems in patients with tinnitus has been well documented (8-10). Herein, tinnitus can cause anxiety, stress, irritability, and depression in the affected individuals. The constant presence of the distressing ringing sounds can be mentally exhausting and affect overall mood and emotional well-being. Additionally, tinnitus can affect social interactions and personal relationships (18). Those suffering from tinnitus might find it challenging to participate in social activities or work in noisy environments.

The co-existence of hearing loss and loudness intolerance problems (i.e., hyperacusis, misophonia and phonophobia) may further complicate the condition (19). It can be challenging to engage in conversations or participate in group settings due to difficulties in hearing or understanding others in the presence of loud and distressing tinnitus. Furthermore, the cognitive abilities patients with tinnitus may also be impacted (20, 21). The prolonged exposure to tinnitus may affect cognitive functions such as memory and information processing. In this regard, the affected patients may experience difficulties in remembering things or maintaining mental clarity. Collectively, to minimize the negative impacts of tinnitus, patients with tinnitus should be properly diagnosed and intervened accordingly.

Teleaudiology

In clinical practice, audiologists are the primary clinicians who play a notable role in evaluating and treating those with tinnitus. Audiology is a service that usually delivers services to patients in a face-to-face setting. Teleaudiology is a type of telehealth in the field of audiology that involves the use of information and communication technology (ICT) tools such as the telephone, videoconferencing, and email to provide audiology services to patients (22). Generally, teleaudiology services offer many notable benefits, and they have been found to save travel time for audiologists (23), and patients (24). In addition, teleaudiology can reduce travel costs (25, 26), improve patient access to services (27-30), as a platform for professional cooperation (31, 32), and as a facility for monitoring hearing aids installation (32, 33).

Previous studies have found that audiologists do not prefer to use teleaudiology in certain clinical tasks, such as hearing assessments, hearing aids fitting for inexperienced users, cochlear implant mapping, and permanent hearing aids adjustment (34, 35). In this matter, concerns were raised about the quality of communication between audiologists and patients, the ability to discuss private matters, and it is hard to build connection with new patients (34).

It is worth noting that only few audiologists have the specific knowledge and equipment to provide services remotely (36). The COVID-19 pandemic had a significant impact on audiology services, and audiologists must develop ways and modify service delivery techniques, including teleaudiology to ensure that audiology services remain operational during the epidemic (37).

Saunders and Roughley (38) conducted a study to investigate changes in audiology service delivery in the United Kingdom during the COVID-19 pandemic and discovered that teleaudiology became the preferred platform for delivering services. In particular, this study found that approximately 30% of people used teleaudiology prior to the COVID-19 restriction, which increased to 98% during the pandemic. This outcome corroborated data showing an increase in the use of telehealth for the provision of medical services, including audiology.

Meanwhile, audiologists believe that teleaudiology can reduce appointment waiting times, increase patient accessibility, decrease travel time, and offer a positive image of audiology services (34). Furthermore, some of them showed a preference for utilizing telaudiology for services such as counselling and auditory rehabilitation, managing appointments, and conducting follow-up consultations for hearing aids (34, 35). This inclination is bolstered by other research indicating that audiologists' preference to utilize teleaudiology is affected by the nature of the service to be delivered. That is, different services may present varying levels of suitability for remote delivery, and this can influence how readily audiologists integrate teleaudiology into their practice (39).

The current literature on teleaudiology (tinnitus)

Managing patients with tinnitus represents a critical audiological service that demands heightened attention, particularly as depression and anxiety associated with the pandemic have been consistently found to have causal connections with the experience of tinnitus (40). The increased psychological distress during such times can exacerbate tinnitus symptoms, necessitating more focused and adapted services to address the needs of those affected. In this regard, healthcare practitioners should be mindful of the complex interplay between tinnitus, stress, depression, and the circumstances brought on by the COVID-19 pandemic. Social isolation and efforts to avoid contracting the virus can contribute to heightened stress and depression, which in turn can exacerbate the severity of tinnitus (41). Nevertheless, there is limited documentation on the relationship between COVID-19 infection and tinnitus. According to the American Tinnitus Association, the stress and sadness associated with social isolation and virus avoidance increase the likelihood of patients developing tinnitus (42).

Telehealth services have experienced a significant growth among healthcare practitioners as a platform to decrease the risk of COVID-19 infection, especially in vulnerable groups including audiology patients (43, 44). With different levels of success, both asynchronous and synchronous telehealth techniques have been applied in the management of individuals who suffer from tinnitus (36, 45).

It is worth mentioning that studies regarding teleaudiology for tinnitus treatment are relatively limited, but the availability of teleaudiology services is expanding (36,46). Even before the pandemic, multiple studies have established the viability of tinnitus therapy delivered by phone, internet, or hard copy teaching materials (45, 47, 48).

Implementing an internet-based cognitive behavioural therapy (iCBT) method for tinnitus treatment into routine healthcare can be a vital first step in increasing access to care for tinnitus patients (49). It has been proven that the use of iCBT can help in the ease of patients' accessibility, thus reducing the severity of tinnitus (50), and improving the quality of life when tinnitus distress and comorbidities (insomnia, depression, hyperacusis, cognitive failures) are lessened (51). In line with this, the progressive tinnitus management (PTM) delivery through teleaudiology was found to produce significantly better outcomes in reducing anxiety and depression than the wait-list method (48). In addition to benefiting tinnitus patients with anxiety and depression, the use of teleaudiology for tinnitus sufferers will effectively spare services for those with more severe problems that require face-to-face treatment, thus leading to an improvement in the audiology service.

Most of the studies did not particularly assess the stakeholder's acceptance of teleaudiology for specific clinical services, especially teleaudiology for tinnitus rehabilitation. Aazh et al. (52) found that besides influencing audiologists' acceptance, the COVID-19 pandemic also enhanced the acceptance of tinnitus patients towards cognitive behavioural therapy (CBT) at the Royal Surrey County Hospital, UK. This hospital often provides face-to-face audiologist-delivered CBT for tinnitus rehabilitation. In this study, patients were offered teleaudiology CBT via video by utilizing a web-based technology during the COVID-19 lockdown (52). The percentage of patients who accepted teleaudiology sessions and the influencing factors were evaluated. It was found that the teleaudiology service was accepted by 80% of the patients. The primary reasons for those who rejected this service were the lack of access to appropriate equipment and the thought that teleaudiology visits would be ineffective. Having a more severe hearing loss in the better ear raised the likelihood of rejecting teleaudiology when compared to having no hearing loss in the better ear. More distressful tinnitus (as measured by the visual analogue scale) increased the likelihood of refusing teleaudiology-based CBT.

Currently, many mobile applications for tinnitus are available (53). In a study by Kutyba et al. (54), the application of the ReSound Tinnitus Relief™ was found to be useful in reducing the severity of tinnitus (as measured by the tinnitus handicap inventory and tinnitus functional index questionnaires). However, some patients never use any tinnitus mobile application due to the lack of awareness (55).

Future directions

In line with the Sustainable Development Goals (SDGs) of the World Health Organization (WHO), i.e., to achieve universal health coverage, including financial risk protection, access to quality essential health-care services and access to safe, effective, quality, and affordable essential medicines and vaccines for all, having the teleaudiology service for managing patients with tinnitus seems essential. This ICT based service offers many benefits to both clinicians and patients. Nevertheless, to ensure the success of its implementation, several factors should be considered. It is imperative, among other things, to evaluate how well teleaudiology is accepted by healthcare practitioners and patients who suffer from tinnitus with different demographic backgrounds. Further research in this area is therefore encouraged.

References

[1] Katz J, Marshall C, English K, Hood L, Tillery KL. Handbook of clinical audiology. Philadelphia: Lippincott Williams Wilkins, 2015.

[2] Romli M, Wan Mohamad WN, Awang MA, Aw CL, Zakaria MN. The clinical value of bilateral bone conduction testing in hearing diagnosis. Indian J Otol 2020;26(3):182-5.

[3] Zuraida Z, Mohd Normani Z, Dinsuhaimi S, Zalina I, Geshina MS. Development of Malay version of vertigo symptom scale (MVVSS) for clinical use. Malaysian J Med Health Sci 2010;6(2):31-9.

[4] Wahab S, Zakaria MN, Sidek D, Abdul Rahman AH, Shah SA, Abdul Wahab NA. Evaluation of auditory hallucinations in patients with schizophrenia: A validation study of the Malay version of Psychotic Symptom Rating Scales (PSYRATS). Psychiatry Res 2015;228(3):462-7.

[5] Abdul Wahab NA, Wahab S, Abdul Rahman AH, Sidek D, Zakaria MN. The hyperactivity of efferent auditory system in patients with schizophrenia: a transient evoked otoacoustic emissions study. Psychiatry Investig 2016;13(1):82-8.

[6] Zakaria MN, Nik Othman NA, Cheu Lih A. Tinnitus severity and the sound therapy outcome. Clin Exp Otorhinolaryngol 2015;8(2):179.

[7] Lih AC, Zakaria MN, Mohamad RA, Nor Rashid MF. Effects of ethnicity and gender on the middle ear function in Asian adults. Indian J Otol 2017;23(2):94-7.

[8] Wan Suhailah WH, Mohd Normani Z, Nik Adilah NO, Azizah O, Aw CL, Zuraida Z. The effectiveness of psychological interventions among tinnitus sufferers: A review. Med J Malaysia 2015;70(3):188-97.

[9] Husain WSW, Othman A, Othman NAN, Mohamad WNW, Zakaria MN. Determining the internal and external reliability of depression, anxiety and stress scales (DASS-21) in assessing psychological symptoms among patients with tinnitus. NeuroQuantology 2018;16(12):67-72.

[10] Shapiro SB, Noij KS, Naples JG, Samy RN. Hearing loss and tinnitus. Med Clin North Am 2021;105(5):799-811.

[11] Wong JW, Wan Mohamad WN, Wan Husain WS, Zakaria MN. The tinnitus suppressive effect: Comparisons between three types of maskers. Int J Disabil Hum Dev 2020;19(1):21-6.

[12] Zakaria MN. The effectiveness of sound therapy in treating patients with mild and severe tinnitus. Int J Disabil Hum Dev 2020;19(2):215-9.

[13] Simonetti P, Vasconcelos LG, Gândara MR, Lezirovitz K, Medeiros ÍRT, Oiticica J. Hearing aid effectiveness on patients with chronic tinnitus and associated hearing loss. Braz J Otorhinolaryngol 2022;88(Suppl 3):S164-70.

[14] Panagiotopoulos NI, Istikoglou CI, Liappas I, Kentroti D, Andreou E, Rizavas I, et al. Cognitive- behavioral psychotherapy of patients with tinnitus. Psychiatriki 2022;33(2):124-38.

[15] Wan Mohamad WN, Hall D, Hoare D, Zakaria MN. Is there a relation between tinnitus severity and hearing handicap? Int J Disabil Hum Dev 2022;21(3):239-44.

[16] Leong SL, Tchen S, Robertson IH, Alsalman O, To WT, Vanneste S. The potential interruptive effect of tinnitus-related distress on attention. Sci Rep 2020;10(1):11911.

[17] Gu H, Kong W, Yin H, Zheng Y. Prevalence of sleep impairment in patients with tinnitus: a systematic review and single-arm meta-analysis. Eur Arch Otorhinolaryngol 2022;279(5):2211-21.

[18] Wang X, Qi M, Zeng X, Cai W, Yin G, Zhang S, et al. Social support and tinnitus distress: the importance of developing positive psychological qualities in patients with chronic tinnitus. Audiol Neurootol 2021;26(4):246-56.

[19] Zakaria MN, Wan Mohamad WN, Rashid MFN, Awang MA, Romli M. Managing a patient with complaints of hearing loss, tinnitus and hyperacusis: Lesson learned. Int J Disabil Hum Dev 2022;21(3):273-7.

[20] Brueggemann P, Neff PKA, Meyer M, Riemer N, Rose M, Mazurek B. On the relationship between tinnitus distress, cognitive performance and aging. Prog Brain Res 2021;262:263-85.

[21] Neff P, Simões J, Psatha S, Nyamaa A, Boecking B, Rausch L, et al. The impact of tinnitus distress on cognition. Sci Rep 2021;11(1):2243.

[22] Jacobs PG, Saunders GH. New opportunities and challenges for teleaudiology within Department of Veterans Affairs. J Rehabil Res Dev 2014;51(5):vii-xii.

[23] Crowell ES, Givens GD, Jones GL, Brechtelsbauer PB, Yao J. Audiology telepractice in a clinical environment: a communication perspective. Ann Otol Rhinol Laryngol 2011;120(7):441-7.

[24] Ramkumar V, Selvakumar K, Vanaja CS, Hall JW, Nagarajan R, Neethi J. Parents' perceptions of tele-audiological testing in a rural hearing screening program in South India. Int J Pediatr Otorhinolaryngol 2016;89:60-6.

[25] Govender SM, Mars M. The use of telehealth services to facilitate audiological management for children: A scoping review and content analysis. J Telemed Telecare 2017;23(3):392-401.

[26] Kokesh J, Ferguson AS, Patricoski C, LeMaster B. Traveling an audiologist to provide otolaryngology care using store-and-forward telemedicine. Telemed J E Health 2009;15(8):758-63.

[27] Coco L, Champlin CA, Eikelboom RH. Community-based intervention determines tele-audiology site candidacy. Am J Audiol 2016;25(3S):264-7.

[28] Edwards M, Stredler-Brown A, Houston KT. Expanding use of telepractice in speech-language pathology and audiology. Volta Rev 2012;112(3):227-42.

[29] Swanepoel de W, Olusanya BO, Mars M. Hearing health-care delivery in sub-Saharan Africa-a role for tele-audiology. J Telemed Telecare 2010;16(2):53-6.

[30] Visagie A, Swanepoel de W, Eikelboom RH. Accuracy of remote hearing assessment in a rural community. Telemed J E Health 2015;21(11):930-7.

[31] Gladden C, Beck L, Chandler D. Tele-audiology: Expanding access to hearing care and enhancing patient connectivity. J Am Acad Audiol 2015;26(9):792-9.

[32] Novak RE, Cantu AG, Zappler A, Coco L, Champlin CA, Novak JC. The future of healthcare delivery: IPE/IPP audiology and nursing student/faculty collaboration to deliver hearing aids vulnerable adults via telehealth. J Nurs Interprofessional Leadersh Qual Saf 2016;1(1):1-13.

[33] Campos PD, Ferrari DV. Teleaudiology: evaluation of teleconsultation efficacy for hearing aid fitting. J Soc Bras Fonoaudiol 2012;24(4):301-8.

[34] Singh G, Pichora-Fuller MK, Malkowski M, Boretzki M, Launer S. A survey of the attitudes of practitioners toward teleaudiology. Int J Audiol 2014;53(12): 850-60.

[35] Kimball SH, Singh G, John AB, Jenstad LM. Implications and attitudes of audiologists towards smartphone integration in hearing healthcare. Hear Res 2018;369:15-23.

[36] Swanepoel de W, Hall JW 3rd. A systematic review of telehealth applications in audiology. Telemed J E Health 2010;16(2):181-200.

[37] Manchaiah V, Eikelboom RH, Bennett RJ, Swanepoel W. International survey of audiologists during the COVID-19 pandemic: effects on the workplace. Int J Audiol 2022;61(4):265-72.

[38] Saunders GH, Roughley A. Audiology in the time of COVID-19: practices and opinions of audiologists in the UK. Int J Audiol 2021;60(4):255-62.

[39] Rashid MFN, Quar TK, Chong FY, Maamor N. Are we ready for teleaudiology?: data from Malaysia. Speech Lang Hear 2020;23(3):146-57.

[40] Beukes E, Ulep AJ, Eubank T, Manchaiah V. The impact of COVID-19 and the pandemic on tinnitus: a systematic review. J Clin Med 2021;10(13):2763.

[41] Narozny W, Tretiakow D, Skorek A. Tinnitus in COVID-19 pandemic. Ear Nose Throat J 2021;100(3_suppl):197S-198S.

[42] Elibol E. Otolaryngological symptoms in COVID-19. Eur Arch Otorhinolaryngol 2021;278(4):1233-6.

[43] Keesara S, Jonas A, Schulman K. COVID-19 and health care's digital revolution. N Engl J Med 2020;382(23):e82.

[44] Swanepoel DW, Hall J. Making audiology work during COVID-19 and beyond. Hear J 2020;73(6):20-4.

[45] Beukes EW, Andersson G, Fagelson M, Manchaiah V. Internet-based audiologist-guided cognitive behavioral therapy for tinnitus: randomized controlled trial. J Med Internet Res 2022;24(2):e27584.

[46] Tao KFM, Brennan-Jones CG, Capobianco-Fava DM, Jayakody DMP, Friedland PL, Swanepoel W, et al. Teleaudiology services for rehabilitation with hearing aids in adults: a systematic review. J Speech Lang Hear Res 2018;61(7):1831-49.

[47] Molini-Avejonas DR, Rondon-Melo S, Amato CA, Samelli AG. A systematic review of the use of telehealth in speech, language and hearing sciences. J Telemed Telecare 2015;21(7):367-76.

[48] Henry JA, Thielman EJ, Zaugg TL, Kaelin C, McMillan GP, Schmidt CJ, et al. Telephone-based progressive tinnitus management for persons with and without traumatic brain injury: a randomized controlled trial. Ear Hear 2019;40(2):227-42.

[49] Weise C, Kleinstäuber M, Andersson G. Internet-delivered cognitive-behavior therapy for tinnitus: a randomized controlled trial. Psychosom Med 2016;78(4):501-10.

[50] Beukes EW, Allen PM, Manchaiah V, Baguley DM, Andersson G. Internet-based intervention for tinnitus: outcome of a single-group open trial. J Am Acad Audiol 2017;28(4):340-51.

[51] Beukes EW, Baguley DM, Allen PM, Manchaiah V, Andersson G. Audiologist-guided internet-based cognitive behavior therapy for adults with tinnitus in the United Kingdom: a randomized controlled trial. Ear Hear 2018;39(3):423-33.

[52] Aazh H, Swanepoel W, Moore BCJ. Telehealth tinnitus therapy during the COVID-19 outbreak in the UK: uptake and related factors. Int J Audiol 2021;60(5):322-7.

[53] Mehdi M, Stach M, Riha C, Neff P, Dode A, Pryss R, et al. Smartphone and mobile health apps for tinnitus: systematic identification, analysis, and assessment. JMIR Mhealth Uhealth 2020;8(8):e21767.

[54] Kutyba J, Gos E, Jędrzejczak WW, Raj-Koziak D, Karpiesz L, Niedziałek I, et al. Effectiveness of tinnitus therapy using a mobile application. Eur Arch Otorhinolaryngol 2022;279(3):1257-67.

[55] Sereda M, Smith S, Newton K, Stockdale D. Mobile apps for management of tinnitus: users' survey, quality assessment, and content analysis. JMIR Mhealth Uhealth 2019;7(1):e10353.

Chapter 7

Exploring the neural basis of tinnitus: Insights into auditory processing mechanisms from auditory brainstem response (ABR) studies

Shamhana A Yusri[1], BSc
Mohd N Zakaria[1], PhD
Nik AN Othman[2], MMed
Cheu L Aw[1], MClinAud
and Wan NW Mohamad[1], PhD

[1]Audiology Programme, School of Health Sciences, Universiti Sains Malaysia, Kelantan, Malaysia
[2]Department of Otorhinolaryngology, School of Medical Sciences, Universiti Sains Malaysia, Kelantan, Malaysia

Abstract

It is evident that many adults with ear problems report the presence of sounds in their ears (even though there are no external sounds). This condition, known as tinnitus, can be serious and requires specialized assessments and dedicated treatments. For many decades, continuous efforts have been made to explain the physiological mechanism of tinnitus. In view of this, the auditory brainstem response (ABR), an electrophysiological assessment, has piqued interest among researchers in order to study the tinnitus generation at the brainstem level. In this chapter, the ABR findings in individuals with tinnitus are reviewed as applicable. It appears that waves I and V of ABR are the useful indicators for describing the possible mechanism of tinnitus generation within the

In: Public Health: Audiology Research in Malaysia
Editors: Mohd N. Zakaria and Joav Merrick
ISBN: 979-8-89530-577-5

brainstem region. Nevertheless, based on the available literature, mixed findings have been reported, in which further research is needed to appropriately understand the tinnitus generation physiologically. In addition, it is also of interest to employ the ABR procedure to study the fundamental aspect of tinnitus suppression physiologically (that underpins the concept of sound therapy), and research in this area is welcomed.

Introduction

Hearing is one of the five senses that allows us to perceive sounds and provides vital information for communication and overall well-being. The external ear, middle ear, inner ear, and central auditory nervous system must be intact so that auditory inputs can be processed and interpreted accordingly (1). Disturbance or damage to any of the components of the hearing system may result in hearing impairment and associated symptoms (2-6).

Tinnitus is one of the common complaints among hearing-impaired individuals (7, 8). It is generally defined as the perception of sound in the absence of a corresponding external auditory stimulus. Individuals with tinnitus often describe the sound that they perceive as buzzing, roaring, clicking or hissing. There are several risk factors and causes that can trigger tinnitus including noise exposure, ototoxic medication, aging, head injury and others (7). It is estimated that around 15% of people have tinnitus, and more than 50 million people in the United States of America suffer from chronic tinnitus (9).

Until the early 1980s, tinnitus was thought to be a cochlear-related phenomenon. However, subsequent research has revealed that tinnitus occurs along the auditory pathway (including the auditory cortex), and patients describe it in a variety of ways, ranging from a single pure tone to a combination of different sounds (10). Even though the exact pathophysiology of tinnitus remains unclear, it is believed that the mechanism responsible for coding tinnitus can originate in the cochlea, the brainstem, or the central nervous system. An increase in spontaneous activity among nerve fibres and more fibres tuned to the same optimal frequency may be linked to the cortical involvement in the tinnitus generation. Individuals experiencing anxiety or emotional reactions to their tinnitus may have involvement in other brain regions. This comprises the amygdala and the autonomic nervous system (11).

Assessment and treatment of tinnitus

It has been well demonstrated that if tinnitus is not treated in a timely manner, many negative consequences will emerge, including psychological disturbances (8, 12). The condition is further worsened in the presence of other comorbid symptoms such as hearing loss and loudness intolerance problems (e.g., hyperacusis, misophonia, and phonophobia) (7, 13, 14).

In clinical practice, hearing healthcare practitioners such as audiologists and otologists will carry out specialized assessments to determine the possible causes of tinnitus, the characteristics of tinnitus, as well as the severity of tinnitus. In addition to the routine audiological assessments, dedicated clinical questionnaires such as the tinnitus handicap inventory (THI), the tinnitus functional index (TFI), and other language-specific questionnaires are administered to obtain insight into how tinnitus affects the daily lives of the affected patients (15-17). Audiologists may perform other assessments, including pitch matching, loudness matching, minimum masking level, and residual inhibition, to acquire information on the features of tinnitus and the tinnitus suppressive effect (18, 19).

In line with the advancement in technology and recent research, various treatment options are now available to decrease the impact of tinnitus on the patients' quality of life (8, 20-26). Hearing aids, tinnitus retraining therapy (TRT), cognitive behavioural therapy (CBT), and sound therapy are among the common treatments for tinnitus. For those who have both hearing loss and tinnitus, the use of hearing aids has been acknowledged as a means of managing both conditions. Hearing aids, which amplify external sounds, have been found to be effective in diverting attention away from and masking the tinnitus (20, 21). The TRT approach, on the other hand, is characterized by a combination of counselling and sound therapy (with white noise as the masker). As demonstrated elsewhere, this intervention method has shown promising results in the management of tinnitus, helping those habituate to the perception of sounds and reduce its impact on their daily lives (22, 23). Meanwhile, the CBT technique employs a concept of counselling, which is a combination of numerous psychological interventions developed and evolved from cognitive and behavioural therapies. This method is effective at relieving tinnitus-related annoyance and improving the patient's emotional state. Although it has no effect on improving the acoustic characteristics of tinnitus, it does improve the response to tinnitus. As such, CBT remains one of the best options for tinnitus treatment (24).

Sound therapy as the tinnitus treatment

In sound therapy, external sounds are presented, aiming to help mask the distressing tinnitus and modify the perception of tinnitus or reaction to it. Many types of noises can be used including white noise, pink noise, music, and others (25, 26).

Even though some noises are better than others, the sound therapy is generally effective in reducing the impacts of tinnitus (25-27). In a meta-analysis study (28), it is confirmed that the sound therapy can significantly reduce the symptom of tinnitus and improve the quality of life. Furthermore, the combination therapies such as TRT, sound stimulation with drug therapy, and sound stimulation with educational consultation have been found to be the most effective treatments for patients with tinnitus (28).

The sound therapy incorporating low-level noises is used to treat individuals with tinnitus based on the tinnitus suppression principle. In a study by Vernon and Meikle (29), 88% of individuals with tinnitus reported some degree of tinnitus suppression. It was also found that the duration of tinnitus suppression varied among individuals with tinnitus, ranging from several seconds to more than 10 minutes. The tinnitus suppressive effect was also dependent on the intensity, duration, and type of stimulus used.

The effectiveness of sound therapy in reducing tinnitus severity has also been demonstrated in other studies (25, 27). In a study by Wong et al. (25), the tinnitus suppressive effect of different auditory stimuli such as white noise (WN), ocean wave (OW), and amplitude modulated (AM) tone was investigated psychophysically among tinnitus patients. When tested with WN, it was discovered that the suppressive effect was evident in all subjects, and WN was deemed the most effective stimulus for tinnitus suppression. Nevertheless, more research efforts are needed to ascertain the current literature on the most optimal stimulus in reducing the impacts of tinnitus.

Auditory brainstem response

When stimulated by repetitive clicks, tone bursts, or even more complex sounds (30-33), the respective action potentials are produced along the auditory system. By having scalp electrodes attached to specific areas of the head, these electrical responses can be recorded and analysed accordingly. The auditory brainstem response (ABR) represents the sum of electrical potentials produced by the specific areas within the brainstem (30). It typically consists of five positive waves (I, II, III, IV, and V). The wave I is believed to be generated by the distal portion of the auditory nerve, while the wave II is evoked by the proximal part of the auditory nerve. The cochlear nucleus is the generator of the wave III, while the wave IV is generated by the superior olivary complex. The most prominent wave of the ABR, i.e., wave V, reflects the electrical responses in the lateral lemniscus and inferior colliculus (30).

The ABR testing has been widely used in clinical practice for many applications. Due to its objective nature, it has been employed for hearing threshold estimation in babies and difficult-to-test children, suspected malingering cases, and medicolegal cases (30). The ABR assessment is commonly used as the site of lesion testing, such as in patients with acoustic neuroma, auditory neuropathy, and those with compromised auditory brainstem functions (30). Additionally, there is also an interest in studying the usefulness of the ABR in understanding the mechanism of tinnitus (34-37).

Auditory brainstem response findings in individuals with tinnitus

To investigate the physiological mechanism of tinnitus, auditory electrophysiological tests including ABR and cortical auditory evoked response (CAER) have been employed (34, 35). Even though the ABR testing has been studied in individuals with tinnitus, the current literature is indeed limited. According to Milloy et al. (36), most of the studies used clicks as the stimuli, and waves I and V were found to be useful in studying the tinnitus mechanism. Nonetheless, they concluded that the results were highly variable because the confounding factors of gender, age, and hearing status were not adequately controlled.

Schaette and McAlpine (37) recorded ABR waveforms using click stimuli from 15 females with tinnitus and 18 females as healthy controls. It was found that the wave I amplitude of ABR that represents the auditory nerve function was significantly reduced in the tinnitus group. This implies that the firing rates of auditory nerve fibres are decreased, in line with the reduced neural output from the cochlea. On the other hand, the wave V amplitude of ABR that represents the neural response from the inferior colliculus was found to be comparable between tinnitus and healthy groups. This paves the way for a better understanding of the tinnitus generation. That is, increased synchronous firing rates of auditory neurons in response to reduced afferent input has been proposed as a mechanism of tinnitus perception (37).

Subsequent studies also found that those with tinnitus had reduced amplitude of wave I of the ABR (38-40). On the other hand, other studies revealed no significant difference in the amplitude of wave I between the control and tinnitus groups (41-44). It is worth noting that even though the authors found that the amplitude of wave I did not differ significantly, the tinnitus group did show reduced amplitude of wave I relative to the control group (43, 44). This can be explained by sporadic damage to the inner hair cells, which may not cause hearing loss but can cause reduced amplitude of wave I (44). The amplitude of the wave I can also be influenced by dys-synchrony in the discharge of the auditory nerve fibres or lesser contribution of responsiveness from the auditory nerve (43).

In line with the findings reported by Schaette and McAlpine (37), other studies also found no significant difference in the amplitude of wave V between the tinnitus and control groups (40, 41, 43-45). Nevertheless, Konadath and Manjula (43) stated that, while the amplitude of wave V did not differ significantly between the groups, the tinnitus group produced a lower mean amplitude of wave V. This could be due to reduced excitation of auditory nerve fibres or the presence of peripheral hearing loss above 8 kHz. Meanwhile, despite the lack of statistically significant findings, Nemati et al. (44) observed increased amplitude of wave V in the tinnitus group, which could indicate increased spontaneous activity of neurons in the brainstem. In contrast, different from other studies, Gu et al. (39) found increased amplitude of wave V at intensity levels of 80 dBnHL and 30 dBnHL. The enhanced amplitude may indicate increased activity in spherical bushy cells and neurons that receive spherical bushy cell inputs (39). Collectively, further research is needed to ascertain the status of wave V amplitude in patients with tinnitus.

The absolute latency of wave I was found to be prolonged in patients with tinnitus (46-49). This could be due to the presence of aberrant neural activity within the auditory nerve (47, 48). On the other hand, other studies reported contradictory results, i.e., the latency of wave I was comparable between the tinnitus and control groups (40, 41, 43-45). Meanwhile, in individuals with tinnitus, the absolute latency of wave V was significantly longer in comparison to the control group (46-50). This latency prolongation may indicate some neural abnormality in the lateral lemniscus or the inferior colliculus (48, 50). Other studies, on the contrary, found that the tinnitus and control groups produced absolute latencies of wave V that did not differ significantly (37, 39-

41, 43, 44). Taken together, further research is clearly needed to ascertain the status of waves I and V in patients with tinnitus.

Future directions

Over the years, efforts have been made to understand the physiological mechanism of tinnitus by utilizing electrophysiological tests such as ABR. Collectively, the available literature has demonstrated the usefulness of ABR testing in revealing the possible mechanisms and theories of tinnitus generation. Additionally, since sound therapy is one of the most common approaches for treating those with tinnitus, it is of interest to unveil the fundamental aspect of tinnitus suppression physiologically. Herein, the ABR assessment can be used for this purpose, and research in this area is encouraged.

References

[1] Lih AC, Zakaria MN, Mohamad RA, Nor Rashid MF. Effects of ethnicity and gender on the middle ear function in Asian adults. Indian J Otol 2017;23(2):94-7.

[2] Zakaria MN, Nik Othman NA, Cheu Lih A. Tinnitus severity and the sound therapy outcome. Clin Exp Otorhinolaryngol 2015;8(2):179.

[3] Romli M, Wan Mohamad WN, Awang MA, Aw CL, Zakaria MN. The clinical value of bilateral bone conduction testing in hearing diagnosis. Indian J Otol 2020;26(3):182-5.

[4] Abdul Wahab NA, Wahab S, Abdul Rahman AH, Sidek D, Zakaria MN. The hyperactivity of efferent auditory system in patients with schizophrenia: A transient evoked otoacoustic emissions study. Psychiatry Investig 2016;13(1):82-8.

[5] Wahab S, Zakaria MN, Sidek D, Abdul Rahman AH, Shah SA, Abdul Wahab NA. Evaluation of auditory hallucinations in patients with schizophrenia: A validation study of the Malay version of Psychotic Symptom Rating Scales (PSYRATS). Psychiatry Res 2015;228(3):462-7.

[6] Zuraida Z, Mohd Normani Z, Dinsuhaimi S, Zalina I, Geshina MS. Development of Malay version of vertigo symptom scale (MVVSS) for clinical use. Malaysian J Med Health Sci 2010;6(2):31-9.

[7] Shapiro SB, Noij KS, Naples JG, Samy RN. Hearing loss and tinnitus. Med Clin North Am 2021;105(5):799-811.

[8] Wan Suhailah WH, Mohd Normani Z, Nik Adilah NO, Azizah O, Aw CL, Zuraida Z. The effectiveness of psychological interventions among tinnitus sufferers: A review. Med J Malaysia 2015;70(3):188-97.

[9] Shargorodsky J, Curhan GC, Farwell WR. Prevalence and characteristics of tinnitus among US adults. Am J Med 2010;123(8):711-8.

[10] Stouffer JL, Tyler RS. Characterization of tinnitus by tinnitus patients. J Speech Hear Disord 1990;55(3):439-53.

[11] Tyler RS, Perreau A. Tinnitus treatment: clinical protocols. New York: Thieme Medical Publishers, 2006.

[12] Husain WSW, Othman A, Othman NAN, Mohamad WNW, Zakaria MN. Determining the internal and external reliability of depression, anxiety and stress scales (DASS-21) in assessing psychological symptoms among patients with tinnitus. NeuroQuantology 2018;16(12):67-72.

[13] Wan Mohamad WN, Hall D, Hoare D, Zakaria MN. Is there a relation between tinnitus severity and hearing handicap? Int J Disabil Hum Dev 2022;21(3):239-44.

[14] Zakaria MN, Wan Mohamad WN, Rashid MFN, Awang MA, Romli M. Managing a patient with complaints of hearing loss, tinnitus and hyperacusis: Lesson learned. Int J Disabil Hum Dev 2022;21(3):273-7.

[15] Newman CW, Jacobson GP, Spitzer JB. Development of the Tinnitus Handicap Inventory. Arch Otolaryngol Head Neck Surg 1996;122(2):143-8.

[16] Fackrell K, Hall DA, Barry JG, Hoare DJ. Psychometric properties of the Tinnitus Functional Index (TFI): Assessment in a UK research volunteer population. Hear Res 2016;335:220-35.

[17] Mohd Normani Z, Wan Suhailah WH, Nik Adilah NO. Test-retest reliability and responsiveness of a Malay tinnitus questionnaire. Med J Malaysia 2018;73(1):7-8.

[18] Lau JYJ, Salim R, Aw CL, Mohamad WNW, Zakaria MN. Are tinnitus pitch and tinnitus loudness correlated with the perceived severity of tinnitus? Findings from Malaysian patients with tinnitus. Int J Disabil Hum Dev 2020;19(1):27-32.

[19] Zakaria MN, Mohamad WNW, Othman NAN, Husain WSW, Wahab NAA. Should we provide sound therapy to a patient with tinnitus but with absent residual inhibition? Int J Disabil Hum Dev 2020;19(2):221-4.

[20] Hazell JW, Wood SM, Cooper HR, Stephens SD, Corcoran AL, Coles RR, et al. A clinical study of tinnitus maskers. Br J Audiol 1985;19(2):65-146.

[21] Simonetti P, Vasconcelos LG, Gândara MR, Lezirovitz K, Medeiros ÍRT, Oiticica J. Hearing aid effectiveness on patients with chronic tinnitus and associated hearing loss. Braz J Otorhinolaryngol 2022;88(Suppl 3):S164-S170.

[22] Phillips JS, McFerran D. Tinnitus Retraining Therapy (TRT) for tinnitus. Cochrane Database Syst Rev 2010;2010(3):CD007330.

[23] Cuesta M, Cobo P. Broadband sound equalized by the hearing loss curves as an improved stimulus for tinnitus retraining therapy-a pilot, non-controlled observational study. J Int Adv Otol 2020;16(2):207-12.

[24] Panagiotopoulos NI, Istikoglou CI, Liappas I, Kentroti D, Andreou E, Rizavas I, et al. Cognitive-behavioral psychotherapy of patients with tinnitus. Psychiatriki 2022;33(2):124-38.

[25] Wong JW, Wan Mohamad WN, Wan Husain WS, Zakaria MN. The tinnitus suppressive effect: Comparisons between three types of maskers. Int J Disabil Hum Dev 2020;19(1):21-6.

[26] Stein A, Wunderlich R, Lau P, Engell A, Wollbrink A, Shaykevich A, et al. Clinical trial on tonal tinnitus with tailor-made notched music training. BMC Neurol 2016;16:38.
[27] Zakaria MN. The effectiveness of sound therapy in treating patients with mild and severe tinnitus. Int J Disabil Hum Dev 2020;19(2):215-9.
[28] Liu H, Zhang J, Yang S, Wang X, Zhang W, Li J, et al. Efficacy of sound therapy interventions for tinnitus management: A protocol for systematic review and network meta-analysis. Medicine (Baltimore) 2021;100(41):e27509.
[29] Vernon JA, Meikle MB. Tinnitus: clinical measurement. Otolaryngol Clin North Am 2003;36(2):293-305.
[30] Hall JW. New handbook of auditory evoked responses. Boston, MA: Pearson, 2007.
[31] Zakaria MN, Wahab NAA, Maamor N, Jalaei B, Dzulkarnain AAA. Auditory brainstem response (ABR) findings in males and females with comparable head sizes at supra-threshold and threshold levels. Neurol Psychiatry Brain Res 2019;32:4-7.
[32] Mukari SZS, Umat C, Chan SC, Ali A, Maamor N, Zakaria MN. Effects of age and type of stimulus on the cortical auditory evoked potential in healthy Malaysian children. J Audiol Otol 2020;24(1):35-9.
[33] Jalaei B, Azmi MHAM, Zakaria MN. Gender differences in binaural speech-evoked auditory brainstem response: are they clinically significant? Braz J Otorhinolaryngol 2019;85(4):486-93.
[34] Bramhall NF, Konrad-Martin D, McMillan GP, Griest SE. Auditory brainstem response altered in humans with noise exposure despite normal outer hair cell function. Ear Hear 2017;38(1):e1-e12.
[35] Morse K, Vander Werff KR. Comparison of silent gap in noise cortical auditory evoked potentials in matched tinnitus and no-tinnitus control subjects. Am J Audiol 2019;28(2):260-73.
[36] Milloy V, Fournier P, Benoit D, Noreña A, Koravand A. Auditory brainstem responses in tinnitus: a review of who, how, and what? Front Aging Neurosci 2017;9:237.
[37] Schaette R, McAlpine D. Tinnitus with a normal audiogram: physiological evidence for hidden hearing loss and computational model. J Neurosci 2011;31(38):13452-7.
[38] Ahmadpour T, Toufan R, Pourbakht A, Kamali M. Evaluation of cochlear synaptopathy in tinnitus patients with normal hearing using auditory brainstem response and electrocochleography tests. Aud Vest Res 2022;31(1):4-10.
[39] Gu JW, Herrmann BS, Levine RA, Melcher JR. Brainstem auditory evoked potentials suggest a role for the ventral cochlear nucleus in tinnitus. J Assoc Res Otolaryngol 2012;13(6):819-33.
[40] Song K, Shin SA, Chang DS, Lee HY. Audiometric profiles in patients with normal hearing and bilateral or unilateral tinnitus. Otol Neurotol 2018;39(6):e416-e421.
[41] Chen PY, Liu TC. Within-subject analysis of auditory brain stem responses in adults with unilateral tinnitus. Ear Nose Throat J 2021;100(5_suppl):592S-596S.
[42] Turner K, Moshtaghi O, Saez N, Richardson M, Djalilian H, Zeng FG, et al. Auditory brainstem response wave I amplitude has limited clinical utility in diagnosing tinnitus in humans. Brain Sci 2022;12(2):142.

[43] Konadath S, Manjula P. Auditory brainstem response and late latency response in individuals with tinnitus having normal hearing. Intractable Rare Dis Res 2016;5(4):262-8.

[44] Nemati S, Faghih Habibi A, Panahi R, Pastadast M. Cochlear and brainstem audiologic findings in normal hearing tinnitus subjects in comparison with non-tinnitus control group. Acta Med Iran 2014;52(11):822-6.

[45] Pinkl J, Wilson MJ, Billingsly D, Munguia-Vazquez R. Detailed analysis of high frequency auditory brainstem response in patients with tinnitus: a preliminary study. Int Tinnitus J 2017;21(1):35-43.

[46] Kehrle HM, Granjeiro RC, Sampaio AL, Bezerra R, Almeida VF, Oliveira CA. Comparison of auditory brainstem response results in normal-hearing patients with and without tinnitus. Arch Otolaryngol Head Neck Surg 2008;134(6):647-51.

[47] Majhi SK, Khandelwal K, Shareef M. Auditory brainstem response in patients of tinnitus with sensorineural hearing loss. Indian J Otolaryngol Head Neck Surg 2019;71(Suppl 2):1495-9.

[48] Ravikumar G, Ashok Murthy V. A study of brainstem auditory evoked responses in normal hearing patients with tinnitus. Indian J Otolaryngol Head Neck Surg 2016;68(4):429-33.

[49] Said EA. Electrophysiological differences in sensorineural hearing loss patients with and without problem-tinnitus. Egypt J Otolaryngol 2012;28(1):22-34.

[50] Cartocci G, Attanasio G, Fattapposta F, Locuratolo N, Mannarelli D, Filipo R. An electrophysiological approach to tinnitus interpretation. Int Tinnitus J 2012;17(2):152-7.

Section two: Hearing

Chapter 8

Cervical vestibular evoked myogenic potential (VEMP) to wide-band chirp and tone burst stimuli: A comparative analysis

Mohd N Zakaria[1], PhD
Wan NW Mohamad[1], PhD
and Zuraida Zainun[2], PhD

[1]Audiology Programme, School of Health Sciences, Universiti Sains Malaysia, Kelantan, Malaysia
[2]Department of Neurosciences, School of Medical Sciences, Universiti Sains Malaysia, Kubang Kerian, Kelantan, Malaysia

Abstract

Cervical vestibular evoked myogenic potential (cVEMP) is an electrophysiological test that is able to measure the status of saccule and inferior vestibular nerve objectively. In order to produce robust cVEMP waveforms, 500 Hz tone burst has been the recommended stimulus. Over the years, there has been a growing interest to study cVEMP when recorded with chirp stimuli. Nevertheless, contradictory results have been reported in the literature in which more research is needed to verify the usefulness of the chirp stimuli in recording cVEMP. Thus, the present study was carried out to compare cVEMP results when tested with wide-band chirp and 500 Hz tone burst stimuli. Twenty healthy young adults (aged 20-24 years) were enrolled in this comparative study. The cVEMP testing was carried out according to the recommended protocol. The stimuli were 500 Hz tone burst (6 ms duration) and custom-built wide-band chirp stimulus (100-10,000 Hz, 10 ms duration). The stimuli were presented through insert earphones at an intensity level of 95 dB nHL

In: Public Health: Audiology Research in Malaysia
Editors: Mohd N. Zakaria and Joav Merrick
ISBN: 979-8-89530-577-5

with a 5.1/s repetition rate. Relative to the tone burst stimulus, P1 and N1 latencies were significantly longer for the wide-band chirp stimulus ($p < 0.001$). The wide-band chirp stimulus also produced statistically smaller P1-N1 amplitudes compared to the tone burst stimulus ($p < 0.001$). To conclude, the 500 Hz tone is still the preferred stimulus for recording cVEMP and should be used without a doubt in clinical settings.

Introduction

Intact ear functions contribute to the ability to enjoy communications in a variety of listening environments and to maintain postural balance while performing daily activities (1-5). Generally, the vestibular organs (i.e., three semicircular canals and two otolith organs), in conjunction with the visual and proprioceptive systems, are responsible to maintain sufficient postural control during static or dynamic conditions (1). In particular, utricle and saccule, which are otolith organs, sense a body's linear acceleration and deceleration in relation to the gravity (5). While the anterior, posterior, and lateral semicircular canals (SCCs) perform roles in the dynamic equilibrium, i.e., to maintain body position in reaction to angular (rotational) acceleration or deceleration (1).

Dizziness may occur if the balance system is compromised. Vertigo (a spinning sensation), the subtype of dizziness, is a common symptom in patients with vestibular disorders (1, 6). As reported elsewhere, the untreated vestibular disorders have serious consequences (1). As such, it is imperative to identify potential individuals with this problem so that appropriate treatments can take place in a timely manner. In clinical settings, various assessments are available to diagnose vestibular dysfunctions (1-5). To objectively diagnose the status of saccule and inferior vestibular nerve, cervical evoked myogenic potential (cVEMP) test is commonly carried out (1, 7, 8). On the other hand, ocular vestibular evoked myogenic potential (oVEMP) test is useful to measure the function of utricle and superior vestibular nerve (1, 7, 8). The cVEMP waveform consists of two prominent peaks (P1 and N1) obtained by presenting loud auditory stimuli with specific placement of electrodes including on sternocledoimastoid (SCM) muscle (2). This electrophysiological test has been studied extensively for the past 30 years and significant advancements have been made in this interesting area (1, 2).

Conventionally, low frequency tone burst stimuli (e.g., 500 Hz) have been the stimuli of interest in the cVEMP recording (1, 2). More recently, there has been a growing interest to study cVEMP evoked by chirp stimuli (7-13). It is worth mentioning that the original purpose of the chirp stimuli was to enhance the waveforms of the auditory brainstem response (ABR) (11, 14, 15). The ABR test is an established electrophysiological assessment that has been used for many decades for various clinical applications including objective hearing threshold estimation (16-18). The chirp stimulus can be of wide-band or narrow-band type (2). Wang et al. (9) pioneered a study that compared amplitudes and latencies of cVEMP when tested with click, 500 Hz tone burst and narrow-band chirp stimuli in 30 healthy individuals. They then found that the chirp stimulus produced statistically earlier cVEMP latencies and larger cVEMP amplitudes relative to the other two stimuli. In line with this, Aydin and her colleagues recorded cVEMP and oVEMP from 56 healthy subjects using wide-band chirp (250-10,900 Hz) and 500 Hz tone burst stimuli (8). Likewise, earlier cVEMP latencies and larger cVEMP amplitudes were noted for the chirp stimulus. Nevertheless, contradictory outcomes have been reported in other studies (7, 10, 13). In a study by Ocal et al. (13) involving 50 healthy adults, cVEMP amplitudes produced by the narrow-band chirp stimulus (centred at 500 Hz, 360-720 Hz) were found to be not statistically different from those of the tone burst stimulus. In accord to this, Reddy and her colleagues conducted a study to compare cVEMP and oVEMP results when evoked by 500 Hz tone burst, narrow-band chirp (centred at 500 Hz, 360-720 Hz), wide-band chirp (200-11,000 Hz) and click stimuli in 54 healthy adults (7). As reported, the narrow-band chirp stimulus produced the largest cVEMP amplitudes, while the cVEMP amplitudes produced by the wide-band chirp were significantly smaller than those of the tone burst. Collectively, due to the inconsistent findings, there is a need to ascertain which stimulus produces the best cVEMP responses. As such, the present study was carried out to compare cVEMP results when recorded with wide-band chirp and tone burst stimuli in healthy adults.

Our study

In this comparative study, 20 otologically normal young adults aged 20-24 years were enrolled. Their hearing status was confirmed with routine clinical assessments, i.e., pure tone audiometry (PTA) and tympanometry (19, 20). In particular, all subjects had hearing thresholds ≤ 20 dB HL (from 250 to

8000 Hz) with a normal middle ear function bilaterally (i.e., type A tympanogram). None of them complained of any symptoms related to vestibular dysfunctions. Each of them signed a consent form declaring that they were willing subjects in the study.

The Biologic auditory evoked potential (AEP) device (Natus Medical Inc., Mundelein, USA) and non-disposable silver disc electrodes were used to record cVEMP waveforms from each participant. For the placement of electrodes, a non-inverting electrode was placed at the midline of the left and right SCM muscles, an inverting electrode was placed on the upper sternum, and a ground electrode was placed on the forehead. The impedance of electrodes was maintained below 5 kΩ throughout the cVEMP testing.

The wide-band chirp was constructed digitally using a LabVIEW software (National Instruments Corp., Texas, USA). The frequency range was set between 100 and 10,000 Hz with a duration of 10 ms. For the 500 Hz tone burst, the duration was 6 ms (i.e., rise time = 2 ms, plateau time = 2 ms, fall time = 2 ms).

The stimuli were presented using insert earphones (ER-3A, Etymotic Research, Illinois, USA) at a 5.1/s stimulus rate and at an intensity level of 95 dB nHL. The time window was set between -10 ms to 50 ms. While the subject was seated comfortably, his/her head was rotated to the opposite side of the test ear (to contract the SCM muscle). To ensure the adequate muscle contraction, the electromyography (EMG) level was maintained (at a minimum level of around 50 μV) using the visual feedback method. The cVEMP responses were averaged after getting 200 sweeps, amplified 5000 times and filtered at 10-1500 Hz. To achieve good waveform reproducibility, the recording was conducted twice for each stimulus. To minimize any potential bias, the order of stimulus presentation was randomized across the subjects. The cVEMP responses were recorded from both ears. All measurements were carried out in a dedicated soundproof room in Audiology Clinic, University Hospital.

Two experienced researchers were involved in identifying the prominent peaks of cVEMP waveforms. Upon the identification of P1 and N1 peaks, the respective latency and amplitude values were computed for each subject. The data normality was ascertained using the Shapiro-Wilk test. Since the data were found to be normally distributed ($p > 0.05$), the respective parametric test was used for statistical analyses. To compare cVEMP results between left and right ears, a paired t-test was used. This analysis was again employed to compare the cVEMP data between wide-band chirp and 500 Hz tone burst stimuli. The p value of less than 0.05 was considered statistically significant.

Findings

Of 20 subjects, half of them were males. They were all Malay and the mean age was 21.6 ± 1.3 years. Reliable cVEMP waveforms were successfully obtained from all subjects (i.e., 100% response rate). An illustration of a cVEMP response recorded with both stimuli from a representative adult subject is shown in Figure 1 (P1 and NI peaks are clearly indicated).

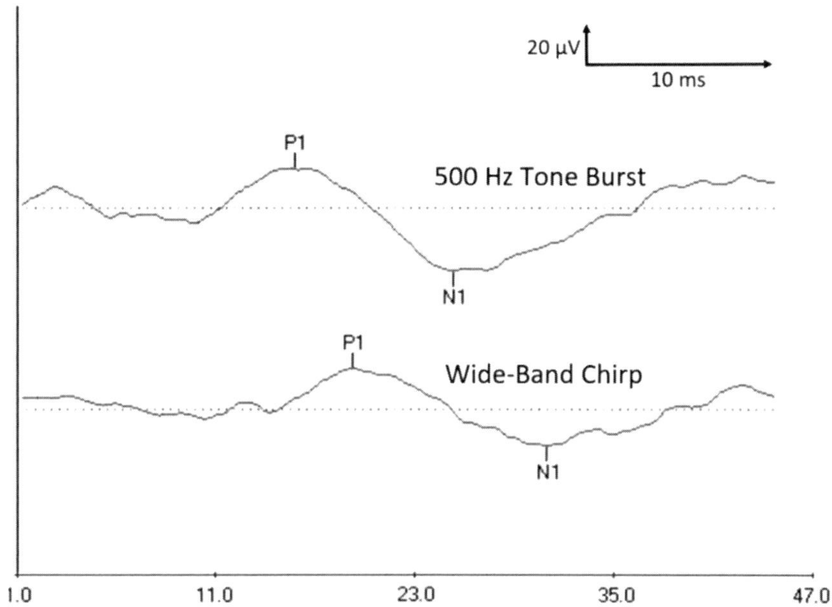

Figure 1. Cervical vestibular evoked myogenic potential (cVEMP) waveforms from a representative adult subject.

Table 1. Mean, standard deviation (SD) and *p* value when cervical vestibular evoked myogenic potential (cVEMP) results are compared between wide-band chirp and 500 Hz tone burst stimuli ($n = 40$ ears)

cVEMP parameter	Wide-band chirp (mean ± SD)	500 Hz tone burst (mean ± SD)	p value
P1 latency (ms)	16.72 ± 3.10	15.08 ± 3.01	< 0.001*
N1 latency (ms)	25.12 ± 3.01	23.29 ± 3.29	< 0.001*
P1-N1 amplitude (µV)	42.96 ± 20.89	68.34 ± 33.18	< 0.001*

*Significant at $p < 0.05$.

Since cVEMP results between left and right ears were found to be not statistically different ($p > 0.05$), these data were then pooled ($n = 40$ ears). Table 1 shows mean, standard deviation (SD) and statistical result (p value) when cVEMP parameters were compared between the wide-chirp and the 500 Hz tone burst stimuli. As revealed, the wide-chirp stimulus produced significantly longer P1 and N1 latencies ($p < 0.001$) compared to the tone burst. Moreover, a statistically smaller mean P1-N1 amplitude was noted for the wide-band chirp stimulus (42.96 ± 20.89 μV) relative to the tone burst (68.34 ± 33.18 μV) and the resultant statistical result was $t(39) = 4.865$, $p < 0.001$.

Discussion

Due to contradictory findings in the literature, the present study was conducted to verify the role of the wide-band chirp in the cVEMP testing. Consistent with the previous reports (7, 9), the response rate of each of cVEMP parameters found in the present study was high (i.e., 100%). Having healthy young adults as the subjects might contribute to this high response rate. The cVEMP results (P1 latency, N1 latency and P1-N1 amplitude) obtained in the present study are also in line with those of the previous studies (7, 9).

As demonstrated, when P1 and N1 latencies were compared between the two stimuli, the wide-band chirp stimulus produced significantly longer latencies. This finding is not consistent with the outcomes of the previous studies. That is, most of the studies found shorter P1 and N1 latencies of cVEMP when recorded with the chirp stimuli (7-10, 13). There are at least two possible reasons to explain the discrepancy between the studies. Firstly, the bandwidth of the chirp stimuli (i.e., wide-band versus narrow-band) may contribute to different study outcomes. In the study by Reddy et al. (7), the narrow-band chirp stimulus (centred at 500 Hz) produced statistically shorter P1 and N1 latencies compared to the 500 Hz tone burst. On the other hand, they found that the wide-band chirp stimulus yielded significantly longer P1 and N1 latencies relative to the narrow-band chirp stimulus. Secondly, most of the studies utilized chirp stimuli commercially available with the AEP devices (known as CE-chirp stimuli) (7-10, 13). As highlighted elsewhere, one possible reason as to why shorter cVEMP latencies were noted for the commercially available chirp stimuli was that their latencies were "purposely" made shorter than the tone burst stimulus (11, 21). Recall that in the present study, a custom-built wide-band chirp stimulus was used to record cVEMP responses. The longer cVEMP latencies produced by the chirp stimulus found in the present study (relative to the tone burst) are indeed in line with the study outcomes reported by Walther and Cebulla (12). In their study, a custom-built band limited chirp stimulus (250-1000 Hz) was employed to record cVEMP and oVEMP from healthy adults and those with vestibular neuritis. They then found that the chirp stimulus produced statistically longer cVEMP latencies than the conventional tone burst in the healthy subjects (12).

In the present study, the wide-band chirp stimulus yielded significantly smaller P1-N1 amplitudes relative to the tone burst stimulus. This finding is not consistent with those of previous studies. That is, most of the studies found larger cVEMP amplitudes when recorded with the chirp stimuli (7-9, 12). Nevertheless, in line with the present study's finding, Özgür et al. found that the chirp stimulus that they employed to record cVEMP produced statistically smaller cVEMP amplitudes compared to the tone burst stimulus (10). Likewise, Reddy et al. (7) reported that the P1-N1 amplitudes evoked with the wide-band chirp stimulus were statistically smaller than those of the tone burst stimulus. On the other hand, in the study by Ocal et al. (13), the cVEMP amplitudes were found to be comparable between the two stimuli. Taken together, further research is warranted to ascertain the influence of different types of chirp stimuli on the cVEMP amplitudes.

The present study had several limitations. Firstly, the sample size used was reasonably small ($n = 40$ ears). In this regard, conducting further large-scale research is advantageous to support the outcomes of the present study. Nevertheless, it is worth mentioning that the statistical power of the study was high (> 0.99) indicating that the study outcomes were indeed valid. Secondly, only healthy young adults were recruited as the subjects and perhaps better study outcomes would be obtained if other age groups are tested. Lastly, the cVEMP testing was only carried out on adults with no vestibular dysfunctions. Herein, to fully appreciate the usefulness of the chirp stimuli (in comparison to the tone burst), conducting studies involving patients with vestibular disorders should be the next step.

Conclusion

Collectively, it was found that the cVEMP waveforms produced by the wide-band chirp stimulus were notably less robust compared to those of the conventional 500 Hz tone burst stimulus (at least when testing healthy young adults). In this regard, the 500 Hz tone remains the recommended stimulus to record cVEMP and should be used without a doubt in clinical settings.

Acknowledgments

The authors would like to thank undergraduate students who were involved in this study. The authors are also thankful to the Ministry of Higher Education Malaysia for funding this research under Fundamental Research Grant Scheme (FRGS) with Project Code: FRGS/1/2020/SKK06/USM/02/7. The authors have stated all possible conflicts of interest within this work.

The authors have stated all sources of funding for this work. If this work involved human participants, informed consent was received from each individual. If this work involved human participants, it was conducted in accordance with the 1964 Declaration of Helsinki. If this work involved experiments with humans or animals, it was conducted in accordance with the related institutions' research ethics guidelines.

References

[1] Katz J, Chasin M, English K, Hood L, Tillery KL. Handbook of clinical audiology. Philadelphia, PA: Lippincott Williams Wilkins, 2015.

[2] Abdallatif AMR, Mohamad WNW, Salim R, Sakeri NSM, Dzulkarnain AAA, Zakaria MN. Is it beneficial to have chirp stimuli in vestibular evoked myogenic potential (VEMP) testing? Int J Disabil Hum Dev 2022;21(3):221-7.

[3] Zainun Z, Zakaria MN, Sidek D, Ismail Z. Clinical use of Malay Version of Vertigo Symptom Scale (MVVSS) in patients with peripheral vestibular disorder (PVD). Med J Malaysia 2012;67(4):386-9.

[4] Zuraida Z, Mohd Normani Z, Dinsuhaimi S, Zalina I, Geshina MS. Development of Malay version of vertigo symptom scale (MVVSS) for clinical use. Malaysian J Med Health Sci 2010;6(2):31-9.

[5] Zakaria MN, Salim R, Tahir A, Zainun Z, Mohd Sakeri NS. The influences of age, gender and geometric pattern of visual image on the verticality perception: A subjective visual vertical (SVV) study among Malaysian adults. Clin Otolaryngol 2019;44(2):166-71.

[6] Agrawal Y, Carey JP, Della Santina CC, Schubert MC, Minor LB. Disorders of balance and vestibular function in US adults: data from the National Health and Nutrition Examination Survey, 2001-2004. Arch Intern Med 2009;169:938-44.

[7] Reddy TM, Heinze B, Biagio-de Jager L, Maes L. Cervical and ocular vestibular evoked myogenic potential: A comparison of narrowband chirp, broadband chirp, tone burst and click stimulation. Int J Audiol 2022;26:1-8.
[8] Aydın C, Önay Ö, Tezcan Eİ, Aşkar Z, Özdek A. Comparison of cervical and ocular vestibular-evoked myogenic potential responses between tone burst versus chirp stimulation. Eur Arch Otorhinolaryngol 2022;279(5):2339-43.
[9] Wang BC, Liang Y, Liu XL, Zhao J, Liu YL, Li YF, et al. Comparison of chirp versus click and tone pip stimulation for cervical vestibular evoked myogenic potentials. Eur Arch Otorhinolaryngol 2014;271(12):3139-46.
[10] Özgür A, Çelebi Erdivanlı Ö, Özergin Coşkun Z, Terzi S, Yiğit E, Demirci M, et al. Comparison of tone burst, click and chirp stimulation in vestibular evoked myogenic potential testing in healthy people. J Int Adv Otol 2015;11(1):33-5.
[11] Zakaria MN, Zainun Z, Cheu Lih A. Considerations when analyzing vestibular evoked myogenic potential (VEMP) outcomes elicited by chirp stimulus in healthy participants. J Int Adv Otol 2015;11(3):271-2.
[12] Walther LE, Cebulla M. Band limited chirp stimulation in vestibular evoked myogenic potentials. Eur Arch Otorhinolaryngol 2016;273(10):2983-91.
[13] Ocal FCA, Karacayli C, Coban VK, Satar B. Can narrow band chirp Stimulus shake the throne of 500 Hz tone burst stimulus for cervical vestibular myogenic potentials? J Audiol Otol 2021;25(2):98-103.
[14] Dau T, Wegner O, Mellert V, Kollmeier B. Auditory brainstem responses with optimized chirp signals compensating basilar membrane dispersion. J Acoust Soc Am 2000;107:1530-40.
[15] Elberling C, Don M. A direct approach for the design of chirp stimuli used for the recording of auditory brainstem responses. J Acoust Soc Am 2010;128:2955-64.
[16] Zakaria MN, Jalaei B, Wahab NA. Gender and modulation frequency effects on auditory steady state response (ASSR) thresholds. Eur Arch Otorhinolaryngol 2016;273(2):349-54.
[17] Zakaria MN, Jalaei B, Aw CL, Sidek D. Are speech-evoked auditory brainstem response (speech-ABR) outcomes influenced by ethnicity? Neurol Sci 2016;37(6):943-8.
[18] Jalaei B, Zakaria MN, Mohd Azmi MH, Nik Othman NA, Sidek D. Gender disparities in speech-evoked auditory brainstem response in healthy adults. Ann Otol Rhinol Laryngol 2017;126(4):290-5.
[19] Romli M, Wan Mohamad WN, Awang MA, Aw CL, Zakaria MN. The clinical value of bilateral bone conduction testing in hearing diagnosis. Indian J Otol 2020;26(3):182-5.
[20] Lih AC, Zakaria MN, Mohamad RA, Nor Rashid MF. Effects of ethnicity and gender on the middle ear function in Asian adults. Indian J Otol 2017;23:94-7.
[21] Zakaria MN, Abdallatif AMR, Mohamad WNW, Salim R, Dzulkarnain AAA. Earlier peak latencies may not fully reflect the robustness of cervical vestibular evoked myogenic potential to CE-chirp stimulus. J Audiol Otol 2022;26(2):108-9.

Chapter 9

Exploring cervical vestibular evoked myogenic potential (VEMP) when recorded with downward chirp stimuli of different frequency ranges

Athar MR Abdallatif[1], BSc
Wan NW Mohamad[1], PhD
Rosdan Salim[2], MMed(ORL-HNS)
and Mohd N Zakaria[1], PhD

[1]Audiology Programme, School of Health Sciences, Universiti Sains Malaysia, Kelantan
[2]Department of Otorhinolaryngology Head and Neck Surgery (ORL-HNS), School of Medical Sciences, Universiti Sains Malaysia, Kubang Kerian, Kelantan, Malaysia

Abstract

Clinically, the function of saccule and inferior vestibular can be objectively measured with cervical vestibular evoked myogenic potential (cVEMP). For the past decades, 500 Hz tone burst has been the stimulus of choice when recording cVEMP. Many researchers have recently become interested in the use of chirp stimuli in cVEMP recording, although further research is needed to fully comprehend this. As such, the aim of this chapter was to compare cVEMP results when tested with chirp stimuli with different frequency ranges. In this comparative study, 25 healthy adults aged 22-45 years underwent the cVEMP testing based on the recommended procedure. Two downward chirp stimuli with different frequency ranges (1000-100 Hz versus 1000-500 Hz) were

In: Public Health: Audiology Research in Malaysia
Editors: Mohd N. Zakaria and Joav Merrick
ISBN: 979-8-89530-577-5

studied. The cVEMP results were found to be comparable between left and right ears for both stimuli ($p > 0.05$). The downward chirp stimulus with a wider frequency range (1000-100 Hz) produced significantly shorter P1 and N1 latencies ($p < 0.05$). Compared to the downward chirp stimulus with a narrower frequency range (1000-500 Hz), the downward chirp stimulus (1000-100 Hz) yielded statistically larger P1, N1 and P1-N1 amplitudes ($p < 0.05$). In conclusion, cVEMP responses can be affected by the frequency range of the chirp stimuli. The downward chirp stimulus with the frequency range of 1000-100 Hz is the preferred option when recording cVEMP.

Introduction

Together with information about the body position, the vestibular system also gives a sense of balance, enabling quick movements in reaction to both internal and external forces. The vestibular system is indeed a crucial part of both postural reflexes and eye movements. As such, balance, eye-movement control, and spatial orientation are all impacted if this system is impaired. In particular, those with vestibular dysfunctions might have severe symptoms like vertigo, nausea, a floating sensation, imbalance, and other forms of sickness (1).

In clinical settings, patients with potential vestibular disorders are required to undergo thorough assessments so that an accurate diagnosis can be made. Before the emergence of cervical vestibular evoked myogenic potential (cVEMP) test, it was difficult to assess the function of otolith organ such as saccule. For example, the conventional tests such as Dix-Hallpike test, head impulse test, caloric test and rotary chair test only measure the status of semicircular canals (2-7). By conducting the cVEMP test, the status of saccule and inferior vestibular nerve can be measured in an objective manner (3-5). It consists of two prominent peaks: a positive peak (P1) with latency of around 13 ms, followed by a negative peak (N1) with latency of around 23 ms. Its diagnostic values have been found to be good and extensively studied in subjects Meniere's disease, acoustic neuroma, labyrinthitis, vestibular neuritis and superior canal dehiscence (SCD) (8-13).

Typically, 500 Hz tone burst is used to record cVEMP either in clinical settings or for research purposes (1, 3-5). This is because this stimulus has been proven to produce the most consistent responses with large amplitudes, which is convenient when testing both normal and vestibular disordered subjects (1, 4). Tone bursts at other frequencies (250 Hz, 750 Hz, 1000 Hz, etc.) can also be used to record cVEMP but their amplitudes are typically smaller than those of 500 Hz tone burst (5, 14-16).

Recently, there is a growing interest to study the diagnostic usefulness of cVEMP test when tested with chirp stimuli (17-23). These chirp stimuli were initially developed and studied to improve the waveforms of auditory brainstem response (ABR) (24, 25). In the ABR testing, the mathematically designed chirp stimuli are able to overcome the cochlear traveling wave delay and consequently, bigger responses are obtained (24, 25). Due to enhanced neural synchrony, the ABR amplitudes produced by the chirp stimuli can be twice bigger than the amplitudes produced by the conventional click stimuli. Typically, robust waveforms are characterized by larger amplitudes and shorter latencies (1).

It is worth stating that all published studies on chirp-evoked cVEMP were carried out using the upward chirp stimuli, i.e., the frequencies are arranged from low to high (e.g., 250-1000 Hz) (20). Different from others, Kamarul Hakim and Zakaria developed a novel custom-built downward chirp stimulus (1000-100 Hz, i.e., arranged from high to low frequencies), and its usefulness was studied accordingly (26). Interestingly, the custom-built downward chirp stimulus was found to produce the most optimum cVEMP responses (i.e., the largest amplitudes and shorter latencies) compared to the upward chirp stimulus (100-1000 Hz) and the 500 Hz tone burst among healthy subjects (26). Owing to this, it was of interest to further explore the diagnostic value of cVEMP evoked by the downward chirp stimulus. As such, the aim of this chapter was to compare cVEMP results when tested with downward chirp stimuli with different frequency ranges.

Our study

Twenty-five healthy Malay adults (aged 22 to 45 years) were invited to take part in the present study, which used a comparative research design. Pure tone audiometry revealed that they all had normal hearing bilaterally (i.e., hearing thresholds ≤ 20 dB HL between 250 and 8000 Hz). Tympanometry was used to confirm healthy middle ear function for both ears (i.e., type A tympanogram). They all denied experiencing any vestibular symptoms in the history taking. Each of them acknowledged their willingness to participate in the study by signing the respective consent form. All assessments were carried out in a dedicated soundproof room within the Audiology Clinic, University Hospital.

The chirp stimuli were digitally constructed using the LabVIEW programme (National Instruments Corp., Texas, USA). Different frequency ranges (i.e., 1000-100 Hz and 1000-500 Hz) were used to produce two different types of downward chirp stimuli. The duration for both stimuli was 10 ms. For the cVEMP recording, the Biologic auditory evoked potential (AEP) device (Natus Medical Inc., Mundelein, USA) was used. The non-disposable silver disc electrodes were chosen, with a non-inverting electrode placed at the midline of the left and right sternocleidomastoid (SCM) muscles, an inverting electrode placed on the upper sternum, and a ground electrode placed on the forehead. The impedance of electrodes was kept below 5 kΩ during all cVEMP measurements.

Insert earphones (ER-3A, Etymotic Research, Illinois, USA) were used to deliver the stimuli at 5.1/s stimulus rate and 95 dB nHL intensity level. The time window was set between -10 ms and 50 ms. During the testing, the subject was seated comfortably and had his/her head turned to the side opposite the test ear (to contract the SCM muscle). In this regard, the visual feedback method was used to ensure appropriate muscular contraction (i.e., the electromyography (EMG) level was maintained at a minimum level of 50 μV). After obtaining 200 sweeps, the cVEMP responses were averaged, amplified 5000 times, and filtered at 10-1500 Hz. For each stimulus, the recording was done twice to ensure adequate waveform repeatability. The order of stimulus presentation was randomised among the subjects to reduce any potential bias. The cVEMP responses from both ears were obtained.

The prominent peaks of the cVEMP waveforms were identified by two vestibular experts. When the P1 and N1 peaks were identified, the corresponding latency and amplitude values for each subject were calculated. The Shapiro-Wilk test was used to determine the data distribution. As it was determined that the data were normally distributed ($p > 0.05$), the appropriate parametric test was conducted as applicable. A paired t-test was applied to compare the cVEMP data between left and right ears. This approach was once more used to compare the cVEMP results between the two downward chirp stimuli. A p value of less than 0.05 was regarded as statistically significant.

Findings

The cVEMP responses were able to be obtained successfully from all subjects (mean age = 27.5 ± 7.6 years). Figure 1 shows cVEMP waveforms produced by the two chirp stimuli from a representative subject. As observed, the downward chirp stimulus with a wider frequency range (1000-100 Hz) seemed to produce more robust cVEMP waveforms relative to the downward chirp stimulus with a narrower frequency range (1000-500 Hz).

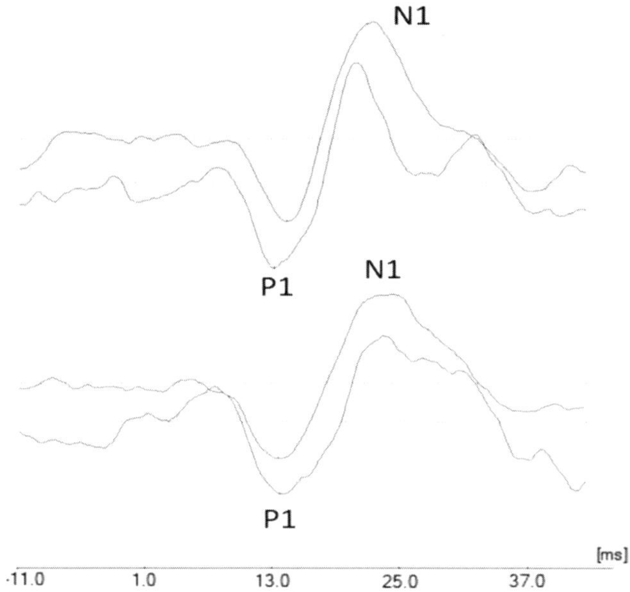

Figure 1. Cervical vestibular evoked myogenic potential (cVEMP) waveforms from a representative adult subject (the upper waveforms and lower waveforms are produced by the downward chirp stimulus (1000-100 Hz) and downward chirp stimulus (1000-500 Hz), respectively).

The paired t-test analysis found the cVEMP results between left and right ears to be comparable for both stimuli ($p > 0.05$). In particular, Tables 1 and 2 show the statistical results for 1000-100 Hz and 1000-500 Hz chirp stimuli, respectively. The cVEMP data were then pooled ($n = 50$ ears) since there were no statistically significant differences between the ears. Table 3 displays the mean, standard deviation (SD), and statistical outcome (p value) when the cVEMP parameters of the two stimuli were compared. As shown, the downward chirp stimulus with a wider frequency range (1000-100 Hz) produced significantly shorter P1 and N1 latencies ($p < 0.05$). Relative to the downward chirp stimulus with a narrower frequency range (1000-500 Hz), the 1000-100 Hz downward chirp stimulus yielded significantly larger P1, N1 and P1-N1 amplitudes ($p < 0.05$).

Table 1. Comparison of cervical vestibular evoked myogenic potential (cVEMP) results between left and right ears for the downward chirp stimulus (1000-100 Hz)

cVEMP parameter	Left ear (mean ± SD)	Right ear (mean ± SD)	p value
P1 latency (ms)	17.0 ± 2.6	17.5 ± 3.0	0.189
N1 latency (ms)	26.3 ± 3.0	26.6 ± 3.2	0.658
P1 amplitude (μV)	54.6 ± 19.8	51.2 ± 21.0	0.471
N1 amplitude (μV)	58.7 ± 25.4	51.6 ± 24.3	0.129
P1-N1 amplitude (μV)	114.0 ± 40.8	104.0 ± 37.0	0.183

Table 2. Comparison of cervical vestibular evoked myogenic potential (cVEMP) results between left and right ears for the downward chirp stimulus (1000-500 Hz)

cVEMP parameter	Left ear (mean ± SD)	Right ear (mean ± SD)	p value
P1 latency (ms)	18.5 ± 3.2	18.4 ± 3.5	0.810
N1 latency (ms)	28.4 ± 2.9	27.9 ± 3.3	0.456
P1 amplitude (μV)	46.4 ± 19.8	44.0 ± 18.0	0.894
N1 amplitude (μV)	47.3 ± 23.3	48.8 ± 21.6	0.810
P1-N1 amplitude (μV)	93.6 ± 38.9	92.8 ± 33.1	0.456

Table 3. Mean, standard deviation (SD) and *p* value when cervical vestibular evoked myogenic potential (cVEMP) results are compared between the two downward chirp stimuli (1000-100 Hz versus 1000-500 Hz)

cVEMP parameter	Chirp (1000-100 Hz) (mean ± SD)	Chirp (1000-500 Hz) (mean ± SD)	p value
P1 latency (ms)	17.3 (2.8)	18.5 (3.3)	0.001*
N1 latency (ms)	26.4 (3.1)	28.2 (3.1)	< 0.001*
P1 amplitude (μV)	52.9 (20.3)	45.2 (18.8)	0.001*
N1 amplitude (μV)	55.1 (24.9)	48.0 (22.2)	0.005*
P1-N1 amplitude (μV)	109.0 (38.9)	93.2 (35.8)	< 0.001*

*Significant at $p < 0.05$.

Discussion

Finding the most optimal stimulus to record cVEMP is essential to produce robust waveforms and beneficial clinically. Even though low frequency tone bursts have been acknowledged as the standard stimuli for recording cVEMP, the potential usefulness of other stimuli (such as chirps) is worthy of investigation. The present study was conducted to determine whether cVEMP responses would be different when evoked by the downward chirp stimuli with different frequency ranges. As stated earlier, reliable cVEMP responses were successfully from all subjects (i.e., 100% response rate). This is in line with the previous studies that also achieved 100% response rate when conducting cVEMP testing with chirp stimuli (17, 21, 22).

The cVEMP results were found to be not statistically different between ears, and this finding was rather expected. In line with the outcomes of other studies (17, 21, 22), symmetrical responses between ears should be obtained when testing healthy subjects. This also suggests that the SCM muscle contraction was adequate and comparable between ears during the cVEMP measurements.

This was the first study to reveal the cVEMP responses elicited by the downward chirp stimuli with different frequency ranges, making comparisons with other studies challenging. Interestingly, the present study found that cVEMP waveforms with shorter latencies and larger amplitudes were produced by the downward chirp stimulus with the 1000-100 Hz frequency range (relative to the 1000-500 Hz chirp stimulus). Given that many studies have demonstrated that tone bursts with frequencies between 500 and 1000 Hz elicit stronger cVEMP responses (5, 14-16), these findings were somewhat unexpected. In this regard, the superiority of the 1000-100 Hz chirp stimulus might be due to its wider frequency range (and therefore, more energy to record cVEMP). It also appears that including frequencies lower than 500 Hz can be advantageous for contributing to more robust cVEMP waveforms. In line with this, many studies have found the chirp stimuli to be better than the conventional 500 Hz tone burst as they produce cVEMP responses with larger amplitudes and shorter latencies (17, 22, 23). Because the chirp stimuli have more energy (e.g., 360-720 Hz for the narrow-band chirp and 250-1000 Hz for the band limited chirp) than the 500 Hz tone burst (20, 22), getting stronger cVEMP responses is therefore possible.

The present study was not without limitations. First, the number of subjects recruited was quite low ($n = 25$). Nevertheless, an attempt was made to increase the statistical power (by combining left and right data resulting in a total of 50 ears), and the study outcomes were indeed sensible. Second, only adults aged between 22 and 45 years were included as the subjects in the present study. In this respect, it can be beneficial to include other age groups for better study outcomes. Finally, the usefulness of the downward chirp stimuli was only studied in a group of healthy subjects. It would be advantageous to also employ these stimuli in the cVEMP testing on those with various vestibular pathologies, and this is subject to further research.

Conclusion

To conclude, the cVEMP latencies and amplitudes are significantly affected by the frequency range of downward stimuli on cVEMP responses. In particular, the downward chirp with a wider frequency range (1000-100 Hz) is the preferred stimulus (relative to the 1000-500 Hz downward chirp stimulus) as it has been found to produce more robust cVEMP waveforms. The stimulus of choice for cVEMP testing in clinical settings, in addition to the conventional 500 Hz tone burst, can be this one.

Acknowledgments

This research was funded by the Ministry of Higher Education Malaysia under Fundamental Research Grant Scheme (FRGS) with Project Code: FRGS/1/2020/SKK06/USM/02/7. The authors have stated all possible conflicts of interest within this work. The authors have stated all sources of funding for this work. If this work involved human participants, informed consent was received from each individual. If this work involved human participants, it was conducted in accordance with the 1964 Declaration of Helsinki. If this work involved experiments with humans or animals, it was conducted in accordance with the related institutions' research ethics guidelines.

References

[1] Katz J, Chasin M, English K, Hood L, Tillery KL. Handbook of clinical audiology. Philadelphia, PA: Lippincott Williams Wilkins, 2015.

[2] Huh YE, Kim JS. Bedside evaluation of dizzy patients. J Clin Neurol 2013;9(4):203-13.

[3] Abdallatif AMR, Mohamad WNW, Salim R, Sakeri NSM, Dzulkarnain AAA, Zakaria MN. Is it beneficial to have chirp stimuli in vestibular evoked myogenic potential (VEMP) testing? Int J Disabil Hum Dev 2022;21(3):221-7.

[4] Rosengren SM, Colebatch JG, Young AS, Govender S, Welgampola MS. Vestibular evoked myogenic potentials in practice: Methods, pitfalls and clinical applications. Clin Neurophysiol Pract 2019;4:47-68.

[5] Zuraida Z, Mohd Normani Z, Din Suhaimi S, Zalina I. Sensitivity and specificity of vestibular evoked myogenic potential elicited by different tone bursts to diagnose peripheral vestibular disordered. Malaysian J Med Health Sci 2014;10(2):9-17.

[6] Zuraida Z, Mohd Normani Z, Dinsuhaimi S, Zalina I, Geshina MS. Development of Malay version of vertigo symptom scale (MVVSS) for clinical use. Malaysian J Med Health Sci 2010;6(2):31-9.

[7] Zakaria MN, Salim R, Tahir A, Zainun Z, Mohd Sakeri NS. The influences of age, gender and geometric pattern of visual image on the verticality perception: A subjective visual vertical (SVV) study among Malaysian adults. Clin Otolaryngol 2019;44(2):166-71.

[8] Dabiri S, Yazdani N, Esfahani M, Tari N, Adil S, Mahvi Z, et al. Analysis of saccular function with vestibular evoked myogenic potential test in Meniere's disease. Acta Med Iran 2017;55(2):123-7.

[9] Chiarovano E, Darlington C, Vidal PP, Lamas G, de Waele C. The role of cervical and ocular vestibular evoked myogenic potentials in the assessment of patients with vestibular schwannomas. PLoS One 2014;9(8):e105026.

[10] Nola G, Guastini L, Crippa B, Deiana M, Mora R, Ralli G. Vestibular evoked myogenic potential in vestibular neuritis. Eur Arch Otorhinolaryngol 2011;268(11):1671-7.

[11] Murofushi T, Halmagyi GM, Yavor RA, Colebatch JG. Absent vestibular evoked myogenic potentials in vestibular neurolabyrinthitis. An indicator of inferior vestibular nerve involvement? Arch Otolaryngol Head Neck Surg 1996;122(8):845-8.

[12] Moon IH, Lee CG, Park MK, Lee JD. Cervical vestibular evoked myogenic potential and ocular vestibular evoked myogenic potential in patients with vestibular neuritis and acute viral labyrinthitis. Res Vest Sci 2012;11(3): 92-6.

[13] Govender S, Fernando T, Dennis DL, Welgampola MS, Colebatch JG. Properties of 500Hz air- and bone-conducted vestibular evoked myogenic potentials (VEMPs) in superior canal dehiscence. Clin Neurophysiol 2016;127(6):2522-31.

[14] Young ED, Fernández C, Goldberg JM. Responses of squirrel monkey vestibular neurons to audio-frequency sound and head vibration. Acta Otolaryngol 1977;84(5-6):352-60.

[15] Janky KL, Shepard N. Vestibular evoked myogenic potential (VEMP) testing: normative threshold response curves and effects of age. J Am Acad Audiol 2009;20(8):514-22.

[16] Piker EG, Jacobson GP, Burkard RF, McCaslin DL, Hood LJ. Effects of age on the tuning of the cVEMP and oVEMP. Ear Hear 2013;34(6):e65-73.

[17] Wang BC, Liang Y, Liu XL, Zhao J, Liu YL, Li YF, et al. Comparison of chirp versus click and tone pip stimulation for cervical vestibular evoked myogenic potentials. Eur Arch Otorhinolaryngol 2014;271(12):3139-46.

[18] Özgür A, Çelebi Erdivanlı Ö, Özergin Coşkun Z, Terzi S, Yiğit E, Demirci M, et al. Comparison of tone burst, click and chirp stimulation in vestibular evoked myogenic potential testing in healthy people. J Int Adv Otol 2015;11(1):33-5.

[19] Zakaria MN, Zainun Z, Cheu Lih A. Considerations when analyzing vestibular evoked myogenic potential (VEMP) outcomes elicited by chirp stimulus in healthy participants. J Int Adv Otol 2015;11(3):271-2.

[20] Walther LE, Cebulla M. Band limited chirp stimulation in vestibular evoked myogenic potentials. Eur Arch Otorhinolaryngol 2016;273(10):2983-91.

[21] Ocal FCA, Karacayli C, Coban VK, Satar B. Can narrow band chirp stimulus shake the throne of 500 Hz tone burst stimulus for cervical vestibular myogenic potentials? J Audiol Otol 2021;25(2):98-103.

[22] Reddy TM, Heinze B, Biagio-de Jager L, Maes L. Cervical and ocular vestibular evoked myogenic potential: A comparison of narrowband chirp, broadband chirp, tone burst and click stimulation. Int J Audiol 2022;26:1-8.

[23] Aydın C, Önay Ö, Tezcan Eİ, Aşkar Z, Özdek A. Comparison of cervical and ocular vestibular-evoked myogenic potential responses between tone burst versus chirp stimulation. Eur Arch Otorhinolaryngol 2022;279(5):2339-43.

[24] Dau T, Wegner O, Mellert V, Kollmeier B. Auditory brainstem responses with optimized chirp signals compensating basilar membrane dispersion. J Acoust Soc Am 2000;107:1530-40.

[25] Elberling C, Don M. A direct approach for the design of chirp stimuli used for the recording of auditory brainstem responses. J Acoust Soc Am 2010;128:2955-64.

[26] Kamarul Hakim S. Vestibular evoked myogenic potential (VEMP) findings in normal individuals using click and chirp stimuli. Dissertation. Kelantan: Universiti Sains Malaysia, 2016.

Chapter 10

The influence of transducer type on the normative values in the sensorineural acuity level (SAL) test

Rosdan Salim[1], MMed(ORL-HNS)
Mahamad A Awang[2], MClinAud
Nik AN Othman[1], MMed(ORL-HNS)
Mohd FN Rashid[2], PhD
and Mohd N Zakaria[2], PhD
[1]Department of Otorhinolaryngology Head and Neck Surgery (ORL-HNS), School of Medical Sciences, Universiti Sains Malaysia, Kubang Kerian, Kelantan, Malaysia
[2]Audiology Programme, School of Health Sciences, Universiti Sains Malaysia, Kelantan, Malaysia

Abstract

Even though pure tone audiometry (PTA) has been widely used for hearing diagnosis in clinical settings, getting masked air conduction (AC) and bone conduction (BC) thresholds can be problematic due to masking problems. To overcome this, the sensorineural acuity level (SAL) test was introduced aiming to estimate the exact BC thresholds which are important in diagnosing the type of hearing loss. Nevertheless, not many studies have been published in determining the clinical usefulness of the SAL test. In this chapter, we aimed to compare the SAL normative data produced by two different transducers (headphones versus insert earphones). Healthy Malaysian adults ($n = 38$) with normal hearing status bilaterally were enrolled in this study. The SAL normative data were

In: Public Health: Audiology Research in Malaysia
Editors: Mohd N. Zakaria and Joav Merrick
ISBN: 979-8-89530-577-5

determined based on the recommended test procedure. It was found that the SAL normative values were comparable when compared between ears at all tested frequencies ($p > 0.05$). Headphones produced statistically higher SAL normative data than insert earphones at the majority of tested frequencies ($p < 0.05$). Collectively, a significant effect of the type of transducer on the SAL normative data was demonstrated in the present study. Our findings can be used accordingly by clinical audiologists, particularly when dealing with masking problems that are commonly encountered in the PTA testing.

Introduction

Having two functioning ears allows humans to enjoy communications while also maintaining postural control in static and dynamic positions (1, 2). Any problems affecting the hearing and vestibular organs may result in notable symptoms such as hearing impairment and vestibular disorder, respectively (1-4). In line with technological advancements, many audiological tests with good diagnostic values are now available to properly diagnose hearing and vestibular disorders (3-8). Early identification and rehabilitation of these disorders are crucial to avoid further negative consequences (9, 10).

Pure tone audiometry (PTA) has been acknowledged as the gold standard test for hearing diagnosis in clinical practice (1). In particular, severity of hearing loss and type of hearing loss can be conveniently determined across frequencies of interest (11,12). By using headphones (or insert earphones), air conduction (AC) thresholds are measured which represent the severity of hearing loss (1). On the other hand, by placing a bone transducer on the mastoid area, bone conduction (BC) thresholds are determined. To determine the type of hearing loss, both AC and BC thresholds are compared (1). Specifically, if the AC thresholds are within the normal range (i.e., ≤ 20 dB HL), BC thresholds are abnormal and significant air-bone gaps (ABGs) are observed (i.e., ≥ 15 dB), a particular patient is said to have conductive hearing loss (CHL) (1). Whereas the occurrence of abnormal AC and BC thresholds (with no significant ABGs) indicates the presence of sensorineural hearing loss (SNHL). The mixed hearing loss (MHL) occurs when both CHL and SNHL are present (1). Getting the exact severity of hearing loss and type of hearing loss is clinically important so that specific treatment options can take place in a timely manner.

In the PTA testing, cross-hearing may occur as the AC transducers tend to vibrate at high intensity levels (i.e., BC pathway is stimulated) (1, 11). In this regard, a continuous masking noise should be given to the non-test ear while presenting the required tonal stimulus to the ear. By doing this, the participation of the non-test ear during the testing can be eliminated, and the exact thresholds can be determined. This masking procedure should be carried out according to the established masking rules (1). Nonetheless, the masking noise delivered to the non-test can be too intense causing a masking problem, known as overmasking (1). When the overmasking phenomenon occurs, obtaining the true thresholds becomes difficult, resulting in an incomplete hearing diagnosis (11, 12).

One of the solutions to obtain valid masked thresholds is to apply a sensorineural acuity level (SAL) test (13-16). This test is particularly useful to estimate masked BC thresholds that are important to confirm the type of hearing loss. In this assessment, a bone vibrator is placed on the forehead, and the masking noise is presented continuously (13). While also wearing headphones (that deliver the pure tone signal), a normally hearing individual is instructed to respond when the tone is heard (in the presence of noise). Herein, AC thresholds in noise are determined for each ear. The SAL normative data are then calculated by computing the differences between AC thresholds in noise and AC thresholds in quiet (by PTA) at the required frequencies (13, 14). Testing more individuals with normal hearing is highly recommended to establish valid SAL normative data (14). When assessing hearing-impaired patients, AC thresholds in noise are obtained at specific frequencies for the ear of interest. The difference between the AC threshold in noise and the SAL normative data is calculated to estimate the respective BC threshold at a specific frequency. As a result, the ABG value will be provided, and since the AC threshold in quiet is known, the BC threshold may now be determined (13).

Despite the fact that the SAL test is useful for overcoming the limitation of PTA testing, not many studies on the SAL test have been reported. More recently, Awang and his colleagues conducted a study to establish SAL normative data among healthy Malaysian participants (15). Their study objective was fulfilled by utilizing insert earphones and two bone transducers (i.e., Radioear B71 and B81). They found that the SAL normative data produced by the two bone vibrators were statistically different at all tested frequencies (15). It is worth noting that no study has been conducted to compare SAL normative values when evaluated with headphones versus insert earphones. Given their different designs, it was hypothesized that the two AC transducers would produce different SAL normative data. Therefore, the present study was conducted to establish SAL normative data by means of headphones and insert earphones, and the comparisons would be made accordingly.

Our study

Thirty-eight healthy Malaysian adults (aged 19 to 47 years) took part in the present study that employed a repeated-measures research design. They all denied having any hearing difficulties in the history taking. The standard PTA testing found them to have normal hearing bilaterally (with hearing thresholds equal to or less than 20 dB HL between 250 and 8000 Hz frequencies). Their middle ear function was also tested and found to be normal bilaterally (i.e., type A tympanogram) (17). Prior to the data collection, each of them signed the respective consent form indicating their willingness to participate in the study voluntarily. All measurements were performed in a soundproof room located in the Audiology Clinic, University Hospital.

Each participant received proper instructions before undergoing the assessments. By using a two-channel audiometer (GSI 61, Grason-Stadler Inc, USA), the PTA testing was carried out primarily to determine AC thresholds in quiet (AC quiet). Meanwhile, the SAL test was carried out to determine AC thresholds in noise (AC noise). TDH-39 headphones (Telephonics, New York, USA) and insert earphones (ER-3A, Etymotic Research, Illinois, USA) were used in the PTA and SAL assessments. The headphones are of the supra-aural type, which rest on the ear but do not entirely enclose the ear, and the insert earphones are made out of a tube that sends pure tones to the ear canal via compressible earplugs.

In the PTA testing, AC thresholds in quiet were determined using the established method (1). In particular, the Hughson-Westlake procedure was employed (i.e., 5dB-up and 10dB-down steps). The AC threshold at a particular frequency was defined when at least two ascending responses were noted (1). The AC thresholds were obtained at frequencies of 250 Hz to 8000 Hz using both transducers. Additionally, BC thresholds (with Radioear B81 bone transducer placed on the mastoid) were also determined (at 250 Hz to 4000 Hz) to ascertain the absence of significant ABGs.

Upon the completion of the PTA testing, the SAL test was conducted in accordance with the procedure proposed by Jerger and Tillman (13). In particular, the B81 bone vibrator was placed on the forehead of the participants, and continuous narrowband sounds were delivered. By placing the AC transducers (headphones and insert earphones in an alternate manner), the respective pure tone signal was presented to either ear. While ignoring the noise, the participants were instructed to only press the response button when the tone was audible. The AC thresholds in noise at frequencies of 250 Hz to 4000 Hz were determined for each ear. For each frequency, the SAL normative values were derived by calculating the differences between AC thresholds in quiet (by PTA) and AC thresholds in noise (by SAL test) (13).

AC thresholds in quite (AC quite), AC thresholds in noise (AC noise) and SAL normative data were computed at all tested frequencies for all participants. The JASP statistical software (version 0.17.1, University of Amsterdam, Netherlands) was used for the data analysis. Both descriptive and inferential statistics were applied accordingly. Since the data were found to be normally distributed ($p > 0.05$ as indicated by the Shapiro-Wilk normality test), the parametric statistical analysis was chosen. In particular, a paired t-test was used to compare the data between left and right ears. This analysis was also utilized to compare the findings between the two AC transducers at the respective test frequencies. A p value of less than 0.05 was set as statistically significant.

Findings

Each of the participants successfully completed the PTA and SAL tests. They were mostly female (65.8%) and had a mean age of 24.4 ± 6.1 years. In terms of ethnicity, the Malay group made up the majority of them (86.8%), followed by the Chinese (13.2%).

The paired t-test analysis found AC quiet, AC noise and SAL normative data between left and right ears to be not statistically different ($p > 0.05$). The data for the left and right ears were then pooled ($n = 76$ ears) to be used in the subsequent analyses. Table 1 displays the mean and standard deviation (SD) of AC thresholds in quiet obtained in the PTA testing. As clearly revealed, both transducers (headphones and insert earphones) produced comparable AC quiet results at all frequencies ($p > 0.05$). The results of AC thresholds in noise (obtained in the SAL test) are shown in Table 2. Descriptively, relative to the insert earphones, the headphones produced higher mean AC noise results at each frequency. This observation was confirmed by the inferential paired t-test analysis, i.e., significant differences were noted in AC noise results between the two transducers ($p < 0.05$). On the other hand, the mean comparisons of SAL normative data are revealed in Table 3. As shown, the headphones produced significantly higher SAL normative data than the insert earphones at frequencies of 250 Hz, 500 Hz, 1000 Hz and 2000 Hz ($p < 0.05$). At 4 kHz, the SAL normative data did not differ statistically ($p = 0.326$).

Table 1. Mean and standard deviation (SD) of air conduction thresholds in quiet obtained using headphones and insert earphones at specific frequencies ($n = 76$ ears), as well as the respective statistical test results

Frequency (Hz)	Transducer	Mean ± SD (dB HL)	p value
250	Headphones	11.8 ± 5.8	0.670
	Insert earphones	11.4 ± 3.9	
500	Headphones	12.4 ± 4.0	0.155
	Insert earphones	13.2 ± 4.4	
1000	Headphones	10.8 ± 5.8	0.101
	Insert earphones	11.9 ± 4.7	
2000	Headphones	9.1 ± 6.2	0.126
	Insert earphones	10.2 ± 5.6	
4000	Headphones	6.4 ± 6.6	0.162
	Insert earphones	5.4 ± 5.9	

Table 2. Mean and standard deviation (SD) of air conduction thresholds in noise obtained using headphones and insert earphones at specific frequencies ($n = 76$ ears), as well as the respective statistical test results

Frequency (Hz)	Transducer	Mean ± SD (dB HL)	p value
250	Headphones	52.1 ± 8.5	< 0.001*
	Insert earphones	44.8 ± 7.5	
500	Headphones	63.2 ± 7.6	< 0.001*
	Insert earphones	58.5 ± 6.6	
1000	Headphones	69.3 ± 6.6	0.023*
	Insert earphones	66.8 ± 7.3	
2000	Headphones	63.2 ± 8.9	0.034*
	Insert earphones	60.8 ± 7.7	
4000	Headphones	57.1 ± 7.2	0.047*
	Insert earphones	54.9 ± 6.9	

*Significant at $p < 0.05$.

Table 3. Mean and standard deviation (SD) of the sensorineural acuity level (SAL) normative data obtained using headphones and insert earphones at specific frequencies ($n = 76$ ears), as well as the respective statistical test results

Frequency (Hz)	Transducer	Mean ± SD (dB)	p value
250	Headphones	40.3 ± 8.8	< 0.001*
	Insert earphones	33.4 ± 7.7	
500	Headphones	50.8 ± 8.6	< 0.001*
	Insert earphones	45.3 ± 7.5	
1000	Headphones	58.5 ± 8.5	0.003*
	Insert earphones	54.9 ± 8.2	
2000	Headphones	54.1 ± 9.4	0.003*
	Insert earphones	50.6 ± 7.9	
4000	Headphones	50.7 ± 8.5	0.326
	Insert earphones	49.6 ± 8.2	

*Significant at $p < 0.05$

Discussion

An alternative assessment is required to determine the exact hearing thresholds because masking problems are frequently encountered during the PTA testing. The SAL test was designed to get around this limitation. Surprisingly, despite the fact that this test was introduced in the 1950s (13), not many studies had been carried out to further explore its clinical usefulness.

The SAL normative data obtained in the present study are nearly similar to those of previous studies (15, 18). Kapoor et al. conducted a study to determine the diagnostic value of the SAL test (in estimating masked BC thresholds) involving healthy participants ($n = 50$) and those with bilateral SNHL ($n = 50$) (18). Similar to the present study, they established the SAL normative values using TDH-39 supra-aural headphones and B81 bone transducer. The reported SAL normative data were 37.5 dB, 50 dB, 58.5 dB, 60 dB and 55 dB at frequencies of 250 Hz, 500 Hz, 1000 Hz, 2000 Hz and 4000 Hz, respectively (18). They also found that the SAL test produced good predictions of the masked BC thresholds at most of the tested frequencies. The SAL normative values reported by other studies were inconsistent with the present study's findings, possibly due to methodological differences between the studies (e.g., different sample sizes, different types of bone vibrators, etc.) (13, 19).

Due to the limited literature, the main aim of the present study was to determine the influence of the type of earphone on the SAL normative values. In clinical practice, headphones are particularly useful when assessing adult patients and those with no ear canal (i.e., canal atresia) (1). On the other hand, insert earphones are advantageous due to higher interaural attenuation values and are more convenient when assessing pediatric patients and those with collapsed ear canals (1,20). As revealed, the SAL normative data produced by the headphones were statistically higher than those of the insert earphones at the majority of the tested frequencies. It is worth mentioning again that the SAL normative were calculated by computing the differences between AC thresholds in quiet and AC thresholds in noise. Based on the results displayed in Table 1, no significant differences in AC thresholds in quiet were noted at all frequencies. These findings are indeed sensible as the output of both transducers are calibrated in dB HL (1). In contrast, the headphones produced significantly higher AC thresholds in noise than the insert earphones at each of frequencies (Table 2). These results were somewhat expected given their different designs. As such, the differences in the SAL normative data produced by the two transducers were likely due to the differences in AC thresholds in noise. In line with this, Awang et al. compared the SAL normative values produced by two bone transducers, i.e., Radioear B71 and B81 (15). They then found that the B71 bone transducer produced significantly higher SAL normative values compared to the B81 bone vibrator. Given that both BC transducers had different designs, getting different SAL normative data was rather expected. Similar to the present study, this study also supports the significant influence of the type of transducer on the SAL normative values (15). Nevertheless, further studies are needed to verify which AC transducer is more useful in estimating BC thresholds when assessing patients with different types of hearing losses.

The present study was not without limitations. Firstly, the sample size employed (n = 38) was modest, and potentially better study results could be attained if more participants were recruited. Keep in mind, however, that in an effort to increase the statistical power and produce the desired study outcomes, the data for the left and right ears were combined (n = 76 ears). Secondly, the present study was limited to participants with normal hearing. As such, it would be advantageous to conduct further research including hearing-impaired groups to ascertain the appropriateness of the SAL normative data collected in this study.

Conclusion

Taken together, the SAL normative values were significantly influenced by the type of transducer. In particular, headphones produced statistically higher SAL normative values than insert earphones at most of the tested frequencies. Because headphones and insert earphones have specific clinical applications (and are equally important), the SAL normative data for both AC transducers are provided by the present study. Clinical audiologists can make appropriate use of these data, particularly when addressing masking problems that are frequently encountered during the PTA testing.

Acknowledgments

This research was funded by the Short Term Grant of Universiti Sains Malaysia with Project Code: 304/PPSK/6315335. The authors have stated all possible conflicts of interest within this work. The authors have stated all sources of funding for this work. If this work involved human participants, informed consent was received from each individual. If this work involved human participants, it was conducted in accordance with the 1964 Declaration of Helsinki. If this work involved experiments with humans or animals, it was conducted in accordance with the related institutions' research ethics guidelines.

References

[1] Katz J, Chasin M, English K, Hood L, Tillery KL. Handbook of clinical audiology. Philadelphia, PA: Lippincott Williams Wilkins, 2015.

[2] Zuraida Z, Mohd Normani Z, Dinsuhaimi S, Zalina I, Geshina MS. Development of Malay version of vertigo symptom scale (MVVSS) for clinical use. Malaysian J Med Health Sci 2010;6(2):31-9.

[3] Zakaria MN, Salim R, Tahir A, Zainun Z, Mohd Sakeri NS. The influences of age, gender and geometric pattern of visual image on the verticality perception: A subjective visual vertical (SVV) study among Malaysian adults. Clin Otolaryngol 2019;44(2):166-71.

[4] Zakaria MN, Zainun Z, Cheu Lih A. Considerations when analyzing vestibular evoked myogenic potential (VEMP) outcomes elicited by chirp stimulus in healthy participants. J Int Adv Otol 2015;11(3):271-2.

[5] Abdul Wahab NA, Wahab S, Abdul Rahman AH, Sidek D, Zakaria MN. The hyperactivity of efferent auditory system in patients with schizophrenia: a transient evoked otoacoustic emissions study. Psychiatry Investig 2016;13(1):82-8.
[6] Zakaria MN, Jalaei B, Wahab NA. Gender and modulation frequency effects on auditory steady state response (ASSR) thresholds. Eur Arch Otorhinolaryngol 2016;273(2):349-54.
[7] Zakaria MN, Jalaei B, Aw CL, Sidek D. Are speech-evoked auditory brainstem response (speech-ABR) outcomes influenced by ethnicity? Neurol Sci 2016;37(6):943-8.
[8] Jalaei B, Zakaria MN, Mohd Azmi MH, Nik Othman NA, Sidek D. Gender disparities in speech-evoked auditory brainstem response in healthy Adults. Ann Otol Rhinol Laryngol 2017;126(4):290-5.
[9] Yoshinaga-Itano C. Benefits of early intervention for children with hearing loss. Otolaryngol Clin North Am 1999;32(6):1089-102.
[10] Sulway S, Whitney SL. Advances in vestibular rehabilitation. Adv Otorhinolaryngol 2019;82:164-9.
[11] Wan Mohamad WN, Romli M, Awang MA, Abdullah R, Lih AC, Zakaria MN. The presence of unusual bone conduction thresholds in pure tone audiometry. Indian J Otol 2020;26(1):54-7.
[12] Romli M, Wan Mohamad WN, Awang MA, Aw CL, Zakaria MN. The clinical value of bilateral bone conduction testing in hearing diagnosis. Indian J Otol 2020;26(3):182-5.
[13] Jerger J, Tillman T. A new method for the clinical determination of sensorineural acuity level (SAL). Arch Otolaryngol 1960; 71: 948-55.
[14] Awang MA, Zakaria MN, Salim R, Rashid MFN. Overcoming masking problems in pure tone audiometry: Better understanding is needed regarding sensorineural acuity level (SAL) test. Int J Disabil Hum Dev 2021;20(1):21-5.
[15] Awang MA, Don AHM, Salim R, Sul'ain MD, Zakaria MN. The normative data for sensorineural acuity level (SAL) test among young adults: comparisons between B71 and B81 bone transducers. Int J Stat Med Res 2021;10:161-8.
[16] Awang MA, Suhaimi MAA, Salim R, Othman NAN, Sul'ain MD, Rashid MFN, et al. Are the normative values of sensorineural acuity level (SAL) test affected by head circumferences of subjects? Int J Stat Med Res 2022;11:169-74.
[17] Lih AC, Zakaria MN, Mohamad RA, Nor Rashid MF. Effects of ethnicity and gender on the middle ear function in Asian adults. Indian J Otol 2017;23(2):94-7.
[18] Kapoor P, Zangmo N, Garg LN, Saini A, Gupta M. Threshold shift validity by documenting sensorineural acuity level: a useful tool for masking. Int J Otorhinolaryngol Head Neck Surg 2020;6(5):913-7.
[19] Goetzinger CP, Porter TA. Study of the sensorineural acuity level test. J Am Audiol Soc 1976;1(4):135-44.
[20] Bess JC. Ear canal collapse: a review. Arch Otolaryngol 1971;93(4):408-12.

Chapter 11

Laryngeal high-speed videoendoscopy: Vocal fold vibratory characteristics of normal speakers

Khairy Anuar Mohd Khairuddin[1,2], MPhil, PhD
Kartini Ahmad[1], MBBCh, PhD
Hasherah Mohd Ibrahim[1], PhD
and Yuling Yan[3], PhD

[1]Speech Sciences Program, Centre for Rehabilitation and Special Needs, Faculty of Health Sciences, Universiti Kebangsaan Malaysia, Kuala Lumpur, Malaysia
[2]Speech Pathology Programme, School of Health Sciences, Universiti Sains Malaysia, Kelantan, Malaysia
[3]Department of Bioengineering, School of Engineering, Santa Clara University, California, United States of America

Abstract

Understanding the vocal fold vibratory characteristics analyzed from laryngeal high-speed videoendoscopy (LHSV) is essential to ensure accurate clinical judgment. Commonly, the LHSV-based analysis methods quantify the glottal area waveform (GAW), extracted from the LHSV images, to generate LHSV-based measures that are applicable in describing the vocal fold vibration. In this chapter we characterize the LHSV-based measures (i.e., $F0_{GAW}$, $jitter_{GAW}$, $shimmer_{GAW}$, OQ_{GAW}, and Nyquist plot) among normal speakers across genders. The participants consisted of 20 normophonic males (mean age of 22.30 ± 1.42) and 36 normophonic females (mean age of 22.28 ± 1.26). Each participant underwent procedures of LHSV to obtain the images of the vocal fold vibration, which were then analyzed to generate the LHSV-based

In: Public Health: Audiology Research in Malaysia
Editors: Mohd N. Zakaria and Joav Merrick
ISBN: 979-8-89530-577-5

measures. Compared to the previous studies, the normal speakers in the present results demonstrated lower $F0_{GAW}$ and $jitter_{GAW}$ but higher OQ_{GAW}. For shimmerGAW, males and females demonstrated lower and higher values, respectively, in comparison to those of the previous findings. In terms of gender-related differences, all quantitative parameters, except for jitterGAW, were found to be different between males and females. Findings of the Nyquist plots revealed that the majority of normal speakers demonstrated the features of broad rim and scattered rim, with comparable distribution across genders. With the use of the current recommended procedures, the study offers more reliable and conclusive findings of the LHSV-based measures of normal speakers across genders. The gender-related differences in most LHSV-based measures suggest that different normative data for males and females are required.

Introduction

A combination of laryngeal high-speed videoendoscopy (LHSV) and image analysis is considered a powerful approach to studying vocal fold vibration (1–3). Several methods have been introduced to analyze images from the LHSV, of which various measures have been used to describe the vocal fold vibratory behaviors (1, 4, 5). One of the LHSV-based analysis methods was developed by Yan et al (1). This analysis method extracts information from the LHSV images to generate the glottal area waveform (GAW), which is then analyzed to produce the LHSV-based measures i.e., quantitative parameters in the forms of GAW-based fundamental frequency ($F0_{GAW}$), glottal perturbation ($jitter_{GAW}$ and $shimmer_{GAW}$), open quotient (OQ_{GAW}), and graphical representation of the vocal fold vibration in the form of the Nyquist plots (1, 6, 7).

Currently, only limited studies reported findings on the characteristics of the LHSV-based measures of normal speakers analyzed from this method (8, 9). These previous studies that were conducted among young American normal speakers used a black and white camera and a recording rate of 2000 frames per second (fps). A summary of the descriptive analyses from these studies is presented in Table 1.

Table 1. Previous findings on the LHSV-based measures of the analysis method by Yan et al. (1)

Participants		Ahmad (9)	Ahmad et al. (8)
		17 males	26 females
Age (Years)	Mean (Range)	26 (19 - 46)	25 (18 - 44)
F0GAW (Hz)	Mean (SD) Range	173 (45) 109 - 273	269 (39) 195 - 375
JitterGAW (%)	Mean (SD) Range	2.4 (0.9) 0.8 - 4.4	1.8 (0.7) 0.9 - 3.6
ShimmerGAW (%)	Mean (SD) Range	3.8 (1.4) 1.9 - 6.8	3.7 (1.3) 1.5 - 7.2
OQGAW	Mean (SD) Range	0.53 (0.11) 0.30 - 0.67	0.71 (0.09) 0.48 - 0.83
Nyquist Plot (%)			
Pattern	I	23	50
	II	71	27
	III	0	15
	IV	6	8

Based on these studies (8, 9), apart from the expected difference in $F0_{GAW}$, findings of the gender-related differences revealed that $jitter_{GAW}$ and $shimmer_{GAW}$ were comparable between males and females. However, OQ_{GAW} was found to be higher in females than that of females. Meanwhile, findings on the Nyquist plots showed that the majority of males and females demonstrated pattern II (i.e., pressed voice vibratory pattern) and pattern I (i.e., clear voice vibratory pattern), respectively, with pattern III (i.e., breathy voice vibratory pattern) was only found among females.

This analysis method has been upgraded to accommodate the advancements in the LHSV technology such as faster recording rate and processing of images from a color high-speed camera, which all were bundled in customized software (10). Accordingly, by incorporating the recommended recording practice in ensuring high quality and reliable LHSV data (11), the measurement protocol for this analysis method has been updated (6, 12) and a more refined interpretation of the Nyquist plots i.e., feature-based classification has been introduced (7). These recent developments demand that the available LHSV-based measures be re-visited to ensure an accurate understanding of the findings using this analysis method. Furthermore, because the previous studies did not involve direct comparison using inferential statistics, the gender-related differences in the LHSV-based measures may benefit from further confirmation.

Understanding the outcomes of the voice evaluation is fundamental to arriving at a valid and reliable clinical decision. With the availability of a range of voice-related measures, even within a similar analytical approach, it is even more critical to be able to accurately interpret the findings. As an example, acoustic analysis, with an array of acoustic measures, necessitates careful interpretation of the findings based on their own specific references to guarantee an accurate conclusion. Similarly, being a relatively recent method of laryngeal visualization that is continuously evolving with the emergence of a variety of new measures and analytical approaches, any LHSV-based analysis method should have specific references for accurate interpretation. Specific to the analysis method by Yan et al. (1), there is a need to update and confirm the available information by adopting the latest recommended recording and analysis protocol.

In this chapter, we aim to characterize the LHSV-based measures among normal speakers. Specifically, the present LHSV-based measures are compared to those of the previous studies to update the currently available findings. These LHSV-based measures are also compared between males and females to examine the gender-related differences, which currently have not been conclusively established. The availability of updated and conclusive information will ensure a valid and reliable interpretation is derived from the evaluation using this analysis method.

Our study

A total of 56 normal speakers, i.e., 20 males and 36 females consisting of undergraduate students of a local university, were recruited via a convenient sampling method as the participants. The mean age of the male and female participants was 22.30 ± 1.42 (a range of 20 to 24 years) and 22.28 ± 1.26 (a range of 21 to 26 years), respectively. Their voices were rated as normal based on the auditory-perceptual rating of voice comprising of a vowel prolongation, a short-voiced sentence production, and a natural conversation. Meanwhile, their vocal folds and larynges were assessed as normal according to the findings of the LHSV recordings. In addition, the participants also did not indicate any significant voice-related issues based on their responses to the medical and voice history questionnaire, which was adapted from Lundy et al. (13). All these components of evaluation were performed by a speech-language therapist with 15 years of specialization in voice pathology. Each participant provided written informed consent to his/her participation following the written and verbal explanations of the study. The conduct of the present study was approved by the university's human ethics committee.

Procedures

The LHSV images of the vocal fold vibration were obtained using the KayPENTAX High-Speed Video System 9710 (Lincoln Park, NJ), which consisted of a color high-speed camera (FASTCAM-MC1; Photron, Tokyo, Japan) attached to a 70-degree rigid endoscope (Model 9106, KayPENTAX, Lincoln Park, NJ) and 300 watts halogen light. The recording rate was set at 4000 fps (14). A spatial resolution of 512 × 256 pixels was used, which was almost similar to the recommended requirement of above 300 × 300 pixels (11).

While in a sitting position, each participant was instructed to open his/her mouth and stick out the tongue. The investigator held the participant's tongue and passed the rigid endoscope orally toward the pharynx until the vocal folds were visible. The participant was asked to phonate a sustained /i/ in a comfortable pitch and loudness. Once the desired view was visualized for at least two seconds, the recording was stopped, and the system automatically stored the video of the final two seconds of the recording, containing about 8000 frames of the images of the vocal fold vibration. The recording was repeated for at least three trials, with five-minute breaks between the trials.

Each successfully recorded video was reviewed using the Photron FASTCAM Viewer (Tokyo, Japan) to identify a portion consisting of the images of the vocal folds in a consistent position and with constant lighting contrast (8). The identified portion was cut, with the unwanted portions discarded. Then, the images in the selected portion were carefully cropped to exclude the unnecessary parts within the frames (e.g., views of the distant structures such as epiglottis and pharyngeal walls). The cropping was carefully done to ensure that the images bordering the vocal folds were amply retained within the frames. For the image analysis, only one video with the best quality in terms of vocal fold position consistency and image lighting contrast was selected from the three trials of each participant. From each video, a segment of interest (SOI) of 2000 frames was selected (6). The customized software performed the analysis to generate the LHSV-based measures.

Images visualizing the complete view of the glottis

A

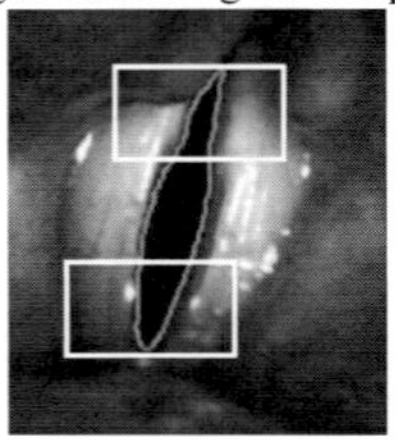

A combination of the fully visible middle glottis and fully visible posterior and anterior glottises (in the white rectangles).

B

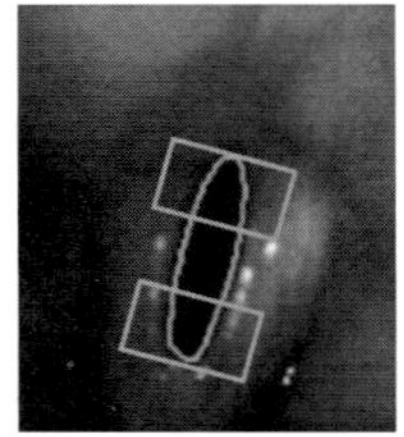

A combination of the fully visible middle glottis and partially visible posterior and anterior glottises with the long tapering of the posterior and anterior glottic outlines (in the blue rectangles).

C

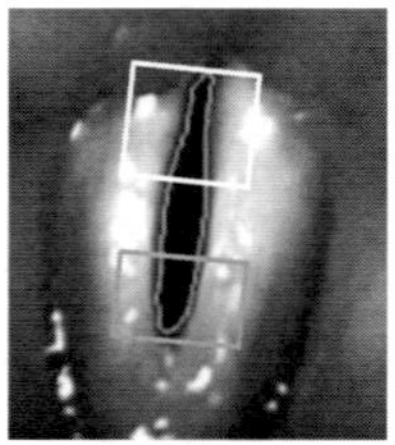

A combination of the fully visible middle glottis and fully visible posterior glottis (in the white rectangle) and partially visible anterior glottis with the long tapering of the anterior glottic outlines (in the blue rectangle).

D

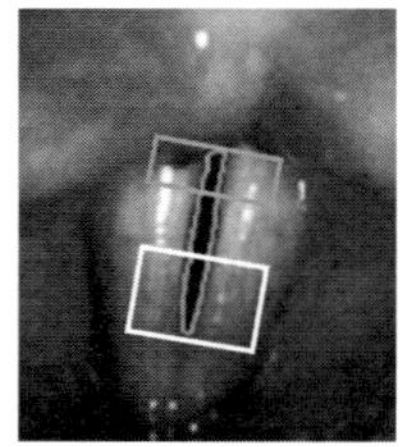

A combination of the fully visible middle glottis and fully visible anterior glottis (in the white rectangle) and partially visible posterior glottis with the long tapering of the posterior glottic outlines (in the blue rectangle).

Images visualizing the posterior-middle view of the glottis

E

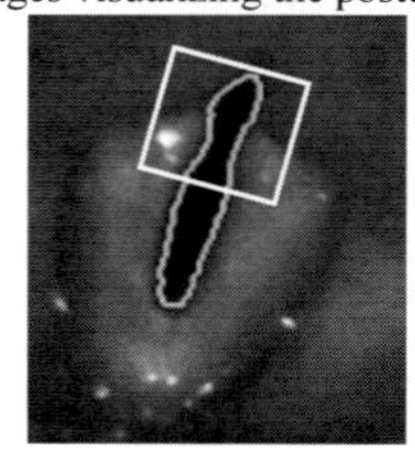

A combination of the fully visible middle glottis and fully visible posterior glottis (in the white rectangle).

F

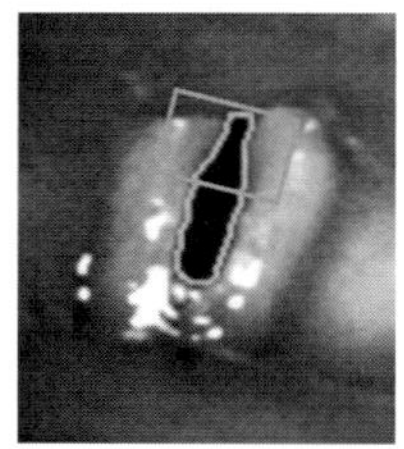

A combination of the fully visible middle glottis and partially visible posterior glottis with the long tapering of the posterior glottic outlines (in the blue rectangle).

Images visualizing the anterior-middle view of the glottis

G

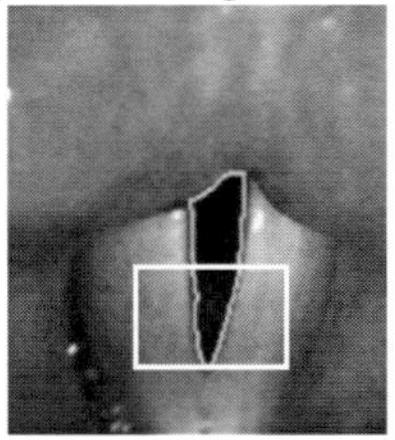

A combination of the fully visible middle glottis and fully visible anterior glottis (in the white rectangle).

H

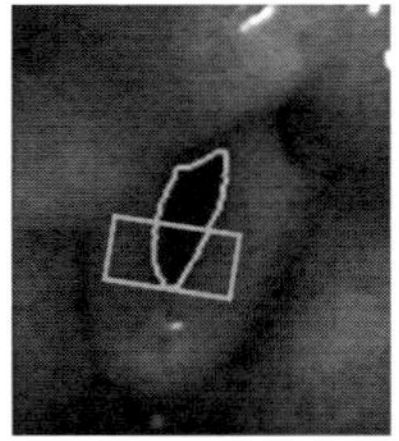

A combination of the fully visible middle glottis and partially visible anterior glottis with the long tapering of the anterior glottic outlines (in the blue rectangle).

Images visualizing the middle view of the glottis

I

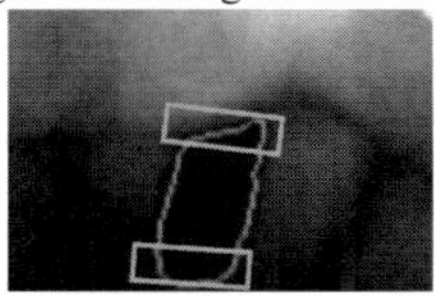

A combination of the fully visible middle glottis and partially visible glottis with the short tapering of the glottic outlines at the posterior or anterior, or both (in the blue rectangles).

Figure 1. Characteristics of the fully and partially visible posterior and anterior glottises.

Analysis of images with partial views of the glottis

Reflecting the situation of the actual clinical practice, not all the obtained images visualized the complete view of the glottis i.e., the whole anterior-posterior length of the vocal folds. It is not uncommon for the visualization of a complete glottis in any laryngeal visualization procedure to be limited by the occlusion of the structures found between the endoscopic camera at the oral-pharyngeal area and the vocal folds (15). Even after employing certain head and neck maneuvers, and body position to improve the visualization, the issue persisted, which resulted in the acquisition of images with a partial view of the glottis.

Given that images visualizing only the anterior-middle and middle views of the glottis affect the OQ_{GAW} (12), the category of views of the glottis depicted in the images was identified and factored into the statistical analysis. The guideline to categorize the views of the glottis is based on the study by Khairuddin (16) and shown in Figure 1.

Statistical analysis

Descriptive statistics such as mean (*M*), standard deviation (*SD*), and range were used to summarize the data. Inferential statistics with the appropriate tests, adhering to the statistical assumptions, were employed to examine the gender-related differences. A significance level of $p < 0.05$ was used for the statistical tests. The effect size was determined according to Cohen (17), of which r of 0.10 = small, 0.30 = medium, 0.50 = large. Meanwhile, for partial eta squared, η_p^2, the effect size was determined based on their corresponding values to d, which 0.01 = small, 0.06 = medium, 0.14 = large (18).

Findings

A descriptive analysis of each quantitative parameter of the male and female groups is shown in Table 2.

A well-known fact of gender difference in fundamental frequency was observed, which suggested that statistical testing to examine the difference in $F0_{GAW}$ was unnecessary. For the other quantitative parameters (see Table 3), the result of a Mann-Whitney *U* test indicated no statistically significant difference in $jitter_{GAW}$ between the groups, with a small effect size of *r*. On the other hand, a statistically significant difference in $shimmer_{GAW}$ was demonstrated between the two groups, which indicated that the group of females showed higher $shimmer_{GAW}$ than that of males, with an *r* approximating a large effect size.

Table 2. Descriptive analyses of all quantitative parameters of the male and female groups

Quantitative parameter	M (SD) Range	
	Males (n = 20)	Females (n = 36)
F0GAW (Hz)	121.93 (18.04) 89 - 158	231.84 (26.77) 193 - 300
JitterGAW (%)	0.58 (0.25) 0.27 - 1.10	0.55 (0.18) 0.21 - 0.91
ShimmerGAW (%)	3.15 (1.34) 1.69 - 7.13	4.68 (1.65) 1.99 - 8.09
OQGAW	0.66 (0.15) 0.44 - 0.93	0.78 (0.13) 0.48 - 0.98

Table 3. Results of a Mann-Whitney *U* test of $jitter_{GAW}$ and $shimmer_{GAW}$ of the male and female groups

Quantitative parameter	Mean Rank		U	z	p	r
	Males	Females				
JitterGAW	28.20	28.67	354.00	-0.103	0.918	0.01
ShimmerGAW	18.78	33.90	165.50	-3.326	0.001*	0.44

*p < 0.05.

Table 4 presents the distribution of the SOIs consisting of images visualizing different views of the glottis, which would be the covariate in the statistical testing of OQ_{GAW}. The result of the analysis of covariance (ANCOVA) revealed a statistically significant difference in OQ_{GAW} between the male and female groups, $F\,(1, 53) = 14.127$, $p < 0.001$, with a large effect size, $\eta_P^2 = 0.21$. This result indicated that the group of females had higher OQ_{GAW} than that of males.

The findings of the Nyquist plots are shown in Table 5. Overall, both groups showed higher percentages of broad rim and scattered rim. According to gender, the male and female groups had comparable percentages of rim width. For rim pattern, only females demonstrated the Nyquist plots with clustered rim.

Table 4. Number and percentage of the SOIs with images visualizing different views of the glottis

View of the glottis	n (%)	
	Males	Females
Complete	11 (55)	12 (33.3)
Posterior-middle	4 (20)	11 (30.6)
Anterior-middle	2 (10)	8 (22.2)
Middle	3 (15)	5 (13.9)

Table 5. Number and percentage of the Nyquist plot features of the male and female groups

Nyquist plot feature		n (%)		
		Males	Females	Total
Rim width				
Narrow	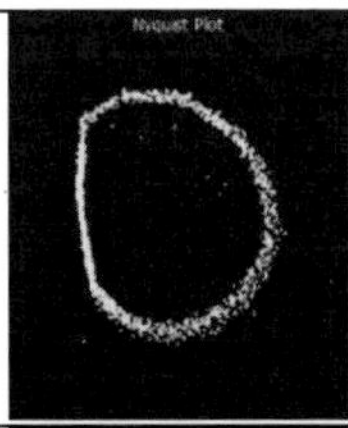	7 (35)	9 (25)	16 (28.6)
Broad	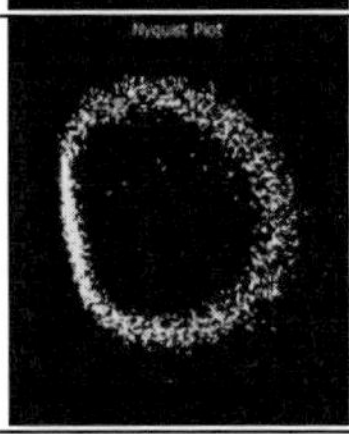	13 (65)	27 (75)	40 (71.4)
	Rim pattern			
Clustered	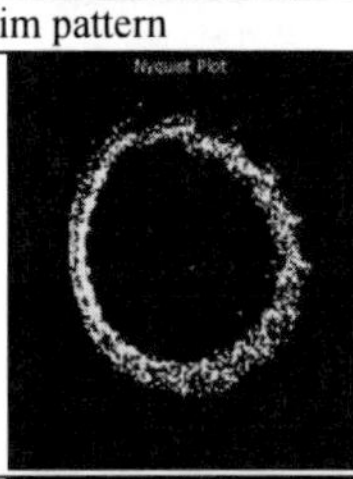	0 (0)	2 (5.6)	2 (3.6)
Scattered	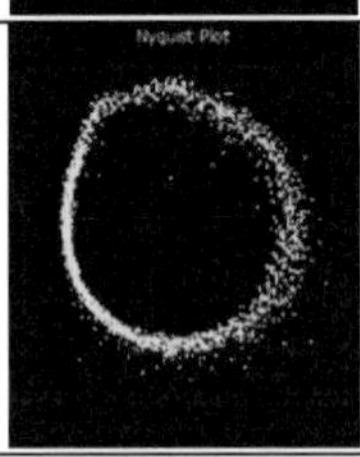	20 (100)	34 (94.4)	54 (96.4)

Discussion

As one of the aims of the present study was to provide an update on the quantitative parameters, the present findings are compared to those of the previous studies (8, 9), which were summarized in Table 1. It was found that the normal speakers in the present study showed lower $F0_{GAW}$ and $jitter_{GAW}$ but higher OQ_{GAW} gender-wise, compared to those of the previous studies. For $shimmer_{GAW}$, varied results were indicated, in which the normal speakers in the present study demonstrated lower and higher $shimmer_{GAW}$ in males and females, respectively, in comparison to those in the findings of the previous studies.

Instead of the differences in the methodology, especially the possible effect of the recording frame rate that is yet to be conclusively confirmed (14), the variation in $F0_{GAW}$ between the present and previous studies may be related to the differences in the characteristics of the sampled populations. In acoustic analysis, descriptive findings revealed that fundamental frequency was lower among young Malaysians (19) compared to young Americans (20), which probably contributed to the differences in vocal tract dimension (21), physiology (20), and linguistics (22) between the two populations. Because they are inherently similar parameters (23), differences in the population characteristics, which explain the variation of the acoustic-based fundamental frequency, are also relevant in understanding the differences of $F0_{GAW}$ between the present and previous studies.

Unlike fundamental frequency, glottal perturbation was clearly shown to be associated with the recording frame rate (24). The study by Schützenberger and colleagues (24) demonstrated that recording rates of 2000 fps and 4000 fps resulted in higher and lower GAW-based jitter, respectively. Therefore, it is suggested that the use of a faster recording rate i.e., 4000 fps, in comparison to a slower recording rate i.e., 2000 fps in the previous studies, resulted in lower $jitter_{GAW}$ in the present results. The differences in the recording frame rate may also explain the finding of lower $shimmer_{GAW}$ among males in the present study. On the other hand, a similar explanation may not be applicable to elucidate the finding of $shimmer_{GAW}$ among females. It is unclear the reason for higher $shimmer_{GAW}$ in the present study than in the previous study among females. However, the larger values of standard deviation and range may indicate the influence of inter-individual variability (25, 26) on this exception in the present finding.

Contrary to glottal perturbation, open quotient was independent of the recording frame rate (24) suggesting that the variations of OQ_{GAW} between the present and previous studies may require a different explanation. A study by Mohd Khairuddin and colleagues (12) found that OQ_{GAW} was greater from the analyses of images visualizing the complete and posterior-middle views of the glottis, especially among those originating from the vocal folds with a posterior glottal gap. Referring to Table 4, the majority of the analyzed images, which depicted the complete and posterior-middle views of the glottis, may lead to higher OQ_{GAW} in the present finding.

Characteristics of the Nyquist plots

Given that the Nyquist plots were interpreted on a different basis i.e., pattern classification in the previous studies (8, 9) and feature-based classification (7) in the present results, an exact comparison may not be meaningful. Nevertheless, similar to the previous studies, as summarized in Table 1, the present results showed that normal speakers adopted different features of the Nyquist plots, indicating varied vibratory behaviors (7). In terms of rim width, the majority of normal speakers demonstrated the Nyquist plots with broad rim. For rim pattern, the Nyquist plots with scattered rim were observed among the majority of normal speakers, but those with clustered rim were only found in a small percentage of females.

The greater occurrence of the Nyquist plots with broad rim and scattered rim, reflecting less regular glottal areas and less regular intra-cycle variations, respectively (7), agrees with the other studies, which also found some amount of irregularity in the majority of normal speakers (27, 28). It is important to note that the irregularity does not constitute a disordered state of vocal fold vibration. Instead, it represents the typical variation, which is common among normal speakers (27). Meanwhile, the findings of only a few normal speakers adopted the Nyquist plots with narrow rim, indicating more regular glottal areas, and clustered rim, signifying more regular intra-cycle variations (7), suggests that only a handful of normal speakers have greater vibratory stability. These ideal vibratory behaviors may be more evident among skillful voice users, such as singers, who are known to have more regular vibratory characteristics (29). Although similar to the previous findings, information from these two features of the Nyquist plots may demonstrate a more reliable conclusion on the regularity measures because they provide condensed data of regularity information derived from a greater number of vibratory cycles (7).

Gender-related differences in the LHSV-based measures

As shown in the results, gender-related differences were found in all quantitative parameters, except for $jitter_{GAW}$. Expectedly, $F0_{GAW}$ were higher in females than males. As a widely accepted fact, this finding does not require further explanation. Similar to the findings of $F0_{GAW}$, females also showed higher $shimmer_{GAW}$ and OQ_{GAW}, in comparison to those males. For the Nyquist plots, although a small percentage of clustered rim was found among females, the overall findings indicated that the distribution of the features of the Nyquist plots was comparable across genders.

Even though they were more varied than the previous studies (8, 9), with the use of inferential statistics, a more conclusive confirmation of the gender-related differences in $jitter_{GAW}$ and $shimmer_{GAW}$ is offered by the present findings. Compared to the other LHSV-based analyses (30, 31), inconsistent trends of glottal perturbation between genders are revealed. These inconsistencies may be related to the inherent discrepancies in the measures quantifying the glottal perturbation (1, 30, 31). The use of various measures to quantify similar behaviors of glottal perturbation has been recognized as one of the issues affecting the comparison of findings between studies, which could be resolved by standardizing the measures to a small set of well-designed parameters (32).

The present findings on OQ_{GAW} between genders are similar to those of the previous studies, as well as the studies that used different types of LHSV-based analyses (30, 31). Granted that they do not differ from those in the literature, with the consideration of the images visualizing different views of the glottis in the analysis, the present result may provide a conclusion that better reflects the actual data in clinical practice. The gender-related differences in OQ_{GAW} are probably related to the presence or absence of the posterior glottal gap. Among females, the consistent presence of the glottic opening originating from the posterior glottal gap would register longer opening phases (8), leading to higher OQ_{GAW}. In contrast, less incidence of posterior glottal gap reduces the presence of the glottic opening, resulting in the detection of shorter opening phases that contribute to lower OQ_{GAW} among males.

For the Nyquist plots, a similar distribution of rim width and rim pattern indicates similar regularity of the glottal areas and the intra-cycle variations, respectively (7), in males and females. Although two females showed the Nyquist plots with clustered rim, the percentage was considered small to clearly differentiate the feature between genders. These findings concur with those of the previous studies that reported no significant differences in vibratory regularity between genders (33, 34).

Conclusion

With the use of the recommended procedures, as well as inferential statistics, it can be assumed that the present findings provide a reliable update of the LHSV-based measures of the normal speakers across genders. The discrepancies in findings between the previous and present studies support the need to make the updated LHSV-based measures available as the latest references. Debatable and even erroneous clinical conclusions may be drawn if the interpretation of findings is based on the previous LHSV-based measures. In addition, confirmation of the presence of gender-related variations in the majority of LHSV-based measures suggests that different databases for males and females are required.

It is acknowledged that the present study is not without limitations. The small sample size and narrow age range may restrict the generalizability of the findings outside the sampled population. Nevertheless, the present findings can be considered valid as a preliminary and additional reference in the interpretation of the LHSV-based measures, particularly using the analysis method by Yan et al. (1), considering the scarcity of similar data.

Acknowledgments

The authors have stated all possible conflicts of interest within this work. The authors have stated all sources of funding for this work. The conduct of this study has been approved by the institution's human ethics committee. Each participant has provided written informed consent after a written and verbal explanation of this study. As this work involved human participants, it was conducted in accordance with the 1964 Declaration of Helsinki.

References

[1] Yan Y, Ahmad K, Kunduk M, Bless D. Analysis of vocal-fold vibrations from high-speed laryngeal images using a Hilbert transform-based methodology. J Voice 2005;19(2):161–75.

[2] Doellinger M. The next step in voice assessment: High-speed digital endoscopy and objective evaluation. Curr Bioinform 2009;4(2):101–11.

[3] Pietruszewska W, Just M, Morawska J, Malinowski J, Hoffman J, Racino A, et al. Comparative analysis of high-speed videolaryngoscopy images and sound data simultaneously acquired from rigid and flexible laryngoscope: A pilot study. Sci Rep 2021;11(1):1–14.

[4] Herbst CT, Herzel H, Švec JG, Wyman MT, Fitch WT. Visualization of system dynamics using phasegrams. J R Soc Interface 2013;10(85):20130288.

[5] Sakakibara KI, Imagawa H, Kimura M, Yokonishi H, Tayama N. Modal analysis of vocal fold vibrations using laryngotopography. In: Proceedings of the 11th Annual Conference of the International Speech Communication Association, Interspeech 2010. Makuhari, Japan; 2010:917–20.

[6] Mohd Khairuddin KA, Ahmad K, Mohd Ibrahim H, Yan Y. Analysis method for laryngeal high-speed videoendoscopy: Development of the criteria for the measurement input. J Voice 2021;35(4):636–45.

[7] Mohd Khairuddin KA, Ahmad K, Mohd Ibrahim H, Yan Y. Description of the features and vibratory behaviors of the Nyquist plot analyzed from laryngeal high-speed videoendoscopy images. J Voice 2022;36(4):582.e11-582.e22.

[8] Ahmad K, Yan Y, Bless DM. Vocal fold vibratory characteristics in normal female speakers from high-speed digital imaging. J Voice 2012;26(2):239–53.

[9] Ahmad K. Laryngeal vibratory characteristics from analysis of high-speed digital images. Doctoral dissertation. Madison, WI: University of Wisconsin-Madison, 2005.

[10] Jiang T, Li G, Luo S, Gu N, Yan Y. Software implementation for the processing of high-speed digital images of the glottis and the analysis of vocal fold vibration. In: Photonic Therapeutics and Diagnostics VIII. San Francisco, California; 2012: 820734.

[11] Deliyski DD. Laryngeal high-speed videoendoscopy. In: Kendall KA, Leonard RJ, eds. Laryngeal evaluation: Indirect laryngoscopy to high-speed digital imaging. New York: Thieme Medical, 2010:245–70.

[12] Mohd Khairuddin KA, Ahmad K, Ibrahim HM, Yan Y. Effects of using laryngeal high-speed videoendoscopy images visualizing partial views of the glottis on measurement outcomes. J Voice 2022;36(1):106–12.

[13] Lundy DS, Roy S, Casiano RR, Xue JW, Evans J. Acoustic analysis of the singing and speaking voice in singing students. J Voice 2000;14(4):490–3.

[14] Deliyski DD, Powell MEG, Zacharias SRC, Gerlach TT, De Alarcon A. Experimental investigation on minimum frame rate requirements of high-speed videoendoscopy for clinical voice assessment. Biomed Signal Process Control 2015;17:21–8.

[15] Verikas A, Uloza V, Bacauskiene M, Gelzinis A, Kelertas E. Advances in laryngeal imaging. Eur Arch Otorhinolaryngol 2009;266(10):1509–20.

[16] Khairuddin KA. Analysis method of laryngeal high-speed videoendoscopy: Development of measurement protocol and application in evaluating vocal fold vibration among different groups of normophonic individuals. Thesis. Kuala Lumpur: Universiti Kebangsaan Malaysia, 2020.

[17] Cohen J. A power primer. Psychol Bull 1992;112(1):155–9.
[18] Fritz CO, Morris PE, Richler JJ. Effect size estimates: Current use, calculations, and interpretation. J Exp Psychol Gen 2012;141(1):2–18.
[19] Ting HN, Chia SY, Abdul Hamid B, Mukari SZMS. Acoustic characteristics of vowels by normal Malaysian Malay young adults. J Voice 2011;25(6):e305–9.
[20] Andrianopoulos M V., Darrow K, Chen J. Multimodal standardization of voice among four multicultural populations formant structures. J Voice 2001;15(1):61–77.
[21] Xue SA, Hao GJP, Mayo R. Volumetric measurements of vocal tracts for male speakers from different races. Clin Linguist Phon 2006;20(9):691–702.
[22] Bahmanbiglu SA, Mojiri F, Abnavi F. The impact of language on voice: An LTAS study. J Voice 2017;31(2):249.e9-249.e12.
[23] Yan Y, Damrose E, Bless D. Functional analysis of voice using simultaneous high-speed imaging and acoustic recordings. J Voice 2007;21(5):604–16.
[24] Schützenberger A, Kunduk M, Döllinger M, Alexiou C, Dubrovskiy D, Semmler M, et al. Laryngeal high-speed videoendoscopy: Sensitivity of objective parameters towards recording frame rate. Biomed Res Int 2016;2016.
[25] Kent RD, Eichhorn JT, Vorperian HK. Acoustic parameters of voice in typically developing children ages 4–19 years. Int J Pediatr Otorhinolaryngol 2021;142:110614.
[26] Brockmann M, Drinnan MJ, Storck C, Carding PN. Reliable jitter and shimmer measurements in voice clinics: The relevance of vowel, gender, vocal intensity, and fundamental frequency effects in a typical clinical task. J Voice 2011;25(1):44–53.
[27] Bonilha HS, Deliyski DD. Period and glottal width irregularities in vocally normal speakers. J Voice 2008;22(6):699–708.
[28] Bonilha HS. Normal vocal fold vibratory amplitude and mucosal wave. In: Kendall KA, Leonard RJ, eds. Laryngeal evaluation. New York: Thieme Medical, 2014: 140–5.
[29] Ravi SK, Shabnam S, George KS, Saraswathi T. Acoustic and aerodynamic characteristics of choral singers. J Voice 2019;33(5):803.e1-803.e5.
[30] Inwald EC, Döllinger M, Schuster M, Eysholdt U, Bohr C. Multiparametric analysis of vocal fold vibrations in healthy and disordered voices in high-speed imaging. J Voice 2011;25(5):576–90.
[31] Patel R, Dubrovskiy D, Döllinger M. Characterizing vibratory kinematics in children and adults with high-speed digital imaging. J Speech Lang Hear Res 2014;57(2):674–86.
[32] Schlegel P, Stingl M, Kunduk M, Kniesburges S, Bohr C, Döllinger M. Dependencies and ill-designed parameters within high-speed videoendoscopy and acoustic signal analysis. J Voice 2019;33(5):811.e1-811.e12.
[33] Choi SH, Choi CH. Qualitative analysis of vocal fold vibration in normal adults with a high-speed video system. Commun Sci Disord 2012;17(4):591–602.
[34] Yamauchi A, Yokonishi H, Imagawa H, Sakakibara KI, Nito T, Tayama N, et al. Age-and gender-related difference of vocal fold vibration and glottal configuration in normal speakers: Analysis with glottal area waveform. J Voice 2014;28(5):525–31.

Chapter 12

The effect of complex auditory stimulations on auditory brainstem response (ABR) in healthy adults

Noor AA Wahab[1], PhD
Suzaily Wahab[2], MMed
Nashrah Maamor[3], PhD
Wan NW Mohamad[4], PhD
and Mohd N Zakaria[4], PhD

[1]Audiology Programme, Centre for Rehabilitation & Special Needs Studies, Faculty of Health Sciences, Universiti Kebangsaan Malaysia, Kuala Lumpur, Malaysia
[2]Department of Psychiatry, Faculty of Medicine, Universiti Kebangsaan Malaysia, Jalan Yaacob Latif, Bandar Tun Razak, Cheras, Kuala Lumpur, Malaysia
[3]Centre for Ear, Hearing and Speech, Faculty of Health Sciences, Universiti Kebangsaan Malaysia, Kuala Lumpur, Malaysia
[4]Audiology Programme, School of Health Sciences, Universiti Sains Malaysia, Kelantan, Malaysia

Abstract

The auditory brainstem response (ABR) test has been used clinically for various applications. Nevertheless, in certain disorders, contradictory results are observed between studies. In view of this, employing complex stimulations in the ABR testing can be beneficial in detecting subtle brainstem problems as well as in assessing the function of binaural hearing. In this chapter, we compare the ABR results when stimulated by monaural and binaural stimulations in the presence of masking noise. In this cross-sectional study, 14 healthy adults (with a mean age of 27.2 ±

In: Public Health: Audiology Research in Malaysia
Editors: Mohd N. Zakaria and Joav Merrick
ISBN: 979-8-89530-577-5

4.1 years) underwent the ABR testing with complex stimulations. The stimuli were custom-built clicks that were mixed with white noise (i.e., simultaneous masking at 0 dB signal to noise ratio). The latencies of waves III and V were found to be significantly shorter in the binaural condition ($p < 0.05$). The binaural stimulation produced a statistically higher mean amplitude of wave V compared to the monaural condition ($p < 0.001$). To conclude, the desired effect of binaural hearing was evident, as the binaural stimulation produced ABR waveforms with statistically shorter latencies and higher amplitudes relative to the monaural stimulation. This complex ABR technique may have the potential to enhance the usefulness of ABR when testing patients with auditory brainstem dysfunctions.

Introduction

The ability of humans to efficiently process acoustic stimuli is dependent on the integrity of auditory systems, which are generally divided into peripheral and central auditory systems (1). The dynamic interaction between these systems plays a significant and diverse role in the processing of incoming acoustic signals. Meanwhile, having two ears is advantageous for improving listening skills for those who have normal hearing. Particularly, the ability to localize sound sources and comprehend conversations in noisy environments is made feasible by this intact binaural hearing (2-4). Anatomically, the binaural hearing advantage is contributed by nerve fibres crossing over between two ears (that start from the superior olivary complex within the auditory brainstem (5). In this regard, depending on the site of the lesion, patients with auditory disorders may have severely impaired binaural hearing, leading to difficulties understanding speech in the presence of noise (1, 4-6).

The auditory evoked potential (AEP) is an objective method for assessing auditory functions (5, 7-10). It is characterized by electrical potentials within the auditory system that are stimulated by repetitive external acoustic stimuli. Upon the stimulation, these electrical responses are picked up by the respective scalp electrodes (placed on specific areas of the head) and visualized on the screen for interpretation (5). The auditory brainstem response (ABR) assessment is a type of AEP that has been widely used in clinical applications for many decades (1, 5). It represents electrical responses derived from specific portions within the auditory brainstem region (5). It consists of five prominent waves (i.e., waves I, II, III, IV, and V) that occur within 5-6 milliseconds after the onset of acoustic stimuli. The waves I and II are generated ipsilaterally by the distal and proximal segments of the auditory nerve, respectively. The wave III is thought to originate from auditory pathways and structures in the pons, including the cochlear nucleus, trapezoid body, and superior olivary complex. The wave IV is generated by multiple brainstem regions, including the superior olivary complex. Meanwhile, the wave V is generated by the lateral lemniscus and inferior colliculus (5).

In clinical practice, the ABR testing has many advantages such as it is not affected by sleeps states, sedation, and anaesthesia (5). It is considered highly valuable clinically because it is non-invasive, does not require active participation from the patient, and provides objective results about the function of the auditory system. Moreover, it has been found to be sensitive in detecting abnormalities within the brainstem region in various pathologies including vestibular schwannoma, brainstem lesions, multiple sclerosis, schizophrenia, and others (5, 6, 11-15). Nevertheless, some studies revealed normal ABR results in participants with suspected brainstem problems (16-18). In view of this, modifications to the routine ABR technique may increase its sensitivity in detecting abnormalities that might exist, and applying more complex stimulations can be beneficial (19). In this chapter, we aim to compare ABR results obtained under monaural and binaural conditions in the presence of noise.

Our study

In this cross-sectional study, 14 healthy volunteers aged 22-36 years agreed to participate. They were selected randomly among students and staff members of the University Hospital. Prior to the ABR testing, all of them underwent pure tone audiometry (PTA) and tympanometry based on the standard clinical protocols (20, 21). Their hearing levels were found to be normal ($\leq$ 20 dB HL at 250 Hz to 8000 Hz) with normal middle ear function (type A tympanogram) for each ear.

The ABR procedure was conducted using a two-channel Biologic Navigator Pro AEP device (Natus Medical Inc., Mundelein, USA) in a dedicated soundproof room in the University Hospital. Adequate instructions were given to each participant prior to the data collection. After cleaning the skin, scalp electrodes were placed on the high forehead (Fpz), forehead (ground), left earlobe (A1) and right earlobe (A2). The impedance between electrodes was maintained below 5 kΩ during the testing.

The stimuli were clicks (250 μs duration) and white noise (with a flat spectrum from 100 Hz to 10,000 Hz) that were custom-built using the Sound Forge Pro software (version 10, Sony, USA). The white noise was then mixed with the custom-built clicks to produce the simultaneous masking effect in the ABR testing (i.e., 0 dB signal to noise ratio). The stimuli used were calibrated in dB nHL.

During the testing, ER-3A insert phones were used to deliver the stimuli at an intensity level of 75 dBnHL with a stimulus rate of 13.3/s. In the monaural stimulation, by randomly selecting the site of the ear, the stimuli were presented ipsilaterally to each ear. Once completed, a 2-minute break was given to the participants before proceeding with the binaural stimulation. In the binaural condition, both ears were stimulated simultaneously.

For each trial, the obtained responses were averaged when 2000 sweeps were obtained. The waveforms were amplified 100,000 times and filtered at 10 Hz to 1500 Hz. The responses were obtained twice for each trial to ensure good test-retest reliability.

Two experienced audiologists (who are the experts in the field of auditory electrophysiology) were involved in confirming the peaks of ABR. Since the data were found to be normally distributed ($p > 0.05$ by the Kolmogorov-Smirnov normality test), the paired t-test was used to compare the ABR results between monaural and binaural stimulations. The p value of less than 0.05 was considered statistically significant. The data analysis was carried out using the MedCalc software (version 20.006, Ostend, Belgium).

Findings

The mean age of the participants involved in this study was 27.2 ± 4.1 years. All of them were Malay, and 50% were females. The prominent peaks of ABR (waves I, III, and V) were present in all participants (i.e., 100% response rate).

Table 1 shows the independent t-test statistical outcomes when the ABR results were compared between monaural and binaural conditions. Descriptively, the absolute latencies of waves I, III, and V were shorter in the binaural stimulation relative to the monaural condition. The t-test analysis then revealed that the latencies of waves III and V were indeed significantly shorter in the binaural condition ($p < 0.05$). While for the ABR amplitudes, a statistically significant result was only obtained when the amplitude of wave V was compared between the two conditions. That is, the binaural stimulation produced a statistically higher mean amplitude of wave V compared to the monaural condition ($p < 0.001$).

Table 1. Comparisons of latencies and amplitudes of waves of auditory brainstem response in monaural and binaural conditions

Parameter	Wave of ABR	Monaural Mean (SD)	Binaural Mean (SD)	P value
Latency (ms)	I	2.60 (0.03)	2.59 (0.06)	0.582
	III	4.74 (0.07)	4.66 (0.07)	0.006*
	V	6.76 (0.17)	6.65 (0.07)	0.034*
Amplitude (μV)	I	0.14 (0.03)	0.18 (0.07)	0.060
	III	0.23 (0.03)	0.21 (0.06)	0.211
	V	0.47 (0.03)	0.65 (0.08)	< 0.001*

*Statistically significant at $p < 0.05$.

Discussion

In the present study, the ABR waveforms were recorded when stimulated by a complex stimulation, i.e., click stimuli in the presence of masking noise (simultaneous masking at 0 dB signal to noise ratio). The aim was to compare the effect of monaural and binaural hearing stimulations in order to determine whether the binaural hearing advantage would be evident.

The latencies of ABR waves obtained in the present study differ from the normative data of ABR to clicks (without masking noise) (5). In particular, the absolutes latencies for both stimulations were longer. As the masking noise may have contributed to the longer latencies, these results were rather expected. Additionally, the study outcomes also support the validity of the simultaneous masking method in the ABR recording (i.e., the masking effect was evident, and the white noise was an effective masker).

As revealed, in the presence of masking noise, the latencies of waves III and V were statistically shorter in the binaural condition. This supports the binaural hearing advantage, i.e., better ABR latencies were observed in the binaural condition than in the monaural stimulation. In this regard, having two functioning ears would be helpful in decreasing the effect of masking (1, 2, 5, 22). Likewise, the binaural condition also elicited ABR waveforms with a higher mean amplitude of wave V, which again supports the existence of binaural hearing effect. It is worth noting that the amplitude of wave III did not differ significantly between the two conditions. In this regard, perhaps better statistical outcomes could be obtained if more participants were recruited. The insignificant statistical results for the amplitude and latency of wave I were rather anticipated, as the cross-over of nerve fibres between the ears does not yet occur at the level of the auditory nerve (5).

There are many pathologies that may compromise the function of the auditory brainstem and binaural hearing (5, 6, 11-15, 23, 24). Schizophrenia, a serious mental illness, is one of the disorders that has piqued interest among researchers (23, 24). While abnormal ABR results were documented in some studies (which suggest abnormal brainstem functions) (13-15), other researchers found normal ABR outcomes when assessing those with schizophrenia (16-18). It is worth stating that many of these studies only employed simple stimulations to record ABR waveforms. In this regard, perhaps better study outcomes could be observed if more complex stimulations (such as in the present study) were employed in the ABR recording.

The present study was not without limitations. First, the sample size used was reasonably small, and perhaps better study outcomes could be obtained if more subjects were involved. Second, this study only recruited normally hearing participants. In view of this, the usefulness of the complex ABR technique (elicited by both monaural and binaural stimulations in noise) should be further supported by including patients with auditory disorders, and this is subject to further research.

Conclusion

The aim of this chapter was to gather physiological evidence regarding the binaural hearing advantage by employing an ABR technique with complex stimulations. The desired effect of binaural hearing was indeed evident, i.e., the binaural stimulation produced ABR waveforms with statistically shorter latencies and higher amplitudes relative to the monaural stimulation. This complex ABR technique may have the potential to increase the sensitivity of ABR when assessing those with compromised auditory brainstem functions.

Acknowledgments

The authors have stated all possible conflicts of interest within this work. The authors have stated all sources of funding for this work. If this work involved human participants, informed consent was received from each individual. If this work involved human participants, it was conducted in accordance with the 1964 Declaration of Helsinki. If this work involved experiments with humans or animals, it was conducted in accordance with the related institutions' research ethics guidelines.

References

[1] Katz J, Chasin M, English K, Hood L, Tillery KL. Handbook of clinical audiology. Philadelphia, PA: Lippincott Williams Wilkins, 2015.

[2] Jalaei B, Azmi MHAM, Zakaria MN. Gender disparity in binaural speech-evoked auditory brainstem response: are they clinically significant? Braz J Otorhinolaryngol 2019;85:486-93.

[3] Boothalingam S, Purcell DW, Allan C, Allen P, Macpherson E. Auditory localization and spatial release from masking in children with suspected auditory processing disorder. Ear Hear 2019;40:1187-96.

[4] Zakaria MN, Wan Mohamad WN, Abdul Wahab NA, Maamor N. Auditory localization performances in subjects with simulated unilateral conductive hearing loss. J Audiol Otol 2018;23:118-9.

[5] Hall JW. New handbook of auditory evoked responses. Boston, MA: Pearson, 2007.

[6] Noffsinger D, Martinez CD, Schaefer AB. Auditory brainstem responses and masking level differences from persons with brainstem lesion. Scand Audiol Suppl 1982;15:81-93.

[7] Mukari SZS, Umat C, Chan SC, Ali A, Maamor N, Zakaria MN. Effects of age and type of stimulus on the cortical auditory evoked potential in healthy Malaysian children. J Audiol Otol 2020;24(1):35-9.

[8] Zakaria MN, Wahab NAA, Maamor N, Jalaei B, Dzulkarnain AAA. Auditory brainstem response (ABR) findings in males and females with comparable head sizes at supra-threshold and threshold levels. Neurol Psychiatry Brain Res 2019;32:4-7.

[9] Zakaria MN, Jalaei B, Aw CL, Sidek D. Are speech-evoked auditory brainstem response (speech-ABR) outcomes influenced by ethnicity? Neurol Sci 2016;37(6):943-8.

[10] Jalaei B, Zakaria MN, Mohd Azmi MH, Nik Othman NA, Sidek D. Gender disparities in speech-evoked auditory brainstem response in healthy adults. Ann Otol Rhinol Laryngol 2017;126(4):290-5.

[11] Koors PD, Thacker LR, Coelho DH. ABR in the diagnosis of vestibular schwannomas: a meta-analysis. Am J Otolaryngol 2013;34(3):195-204.

[12] Rishiq D, Harkrider A, Springer C, Hedrick M. Click-evoked and speech-evoked auditory brainstem responses from individuals with multiple sclerosis. Neurosci Lett 2021;740:135460.

[13] Grillon C, Ameli R, Glazer WM. Brainstem auditory-evoked potentials to different rates and intensities of stimulation in schizophrenics. Biol Psychiatry 1990;28(9):819-23.

[14] Igata M, Ohta M, Hayashida Y, Abe K. Missing peaks in auditory brainstem responses and negative symptoms in schizophrenia. Jpn J Psychiatry Neurol 1994;48(3):571-8.

[15] Källstrand J, Nehlstedt SF, Sköld ML, Nielzén S. Lateral asymmetry and reduced forward masking effect in early brainstem auditory evoked responses in schizophrenia. Psychiatry Res 2012;196(2-3):188-93.

[16] McKay CM, Headlam DM, Copolov DL. Central auditory processing in patients with auditory hallucinations. Am J Psychiatry 2000;157(5):759-66.

[17] Nam EC. Is it necessary to differentiate tinnitus from auditory hallucination in schizophrenic patients? J Laryngol Otol 2005;119(5):352-5.

[18] Clayson PE, Joshi YB, Thomas ML, Sprock J, Nungaray J, Swerdlow NR, et al. Click-evoked auditory brainstem responses (ABRs) are intact in schizophrenia and not sensitive to cognitive training. Biomark Neuropsychiatry 2022;6:100046.

[19] Tarasenko MA, Swerdlow NR, Makeig S, Braff DL, Light GA. The auditory brain-stem response to complex sounds: a potential biomarker for guiding treatment of psychosis. Front Psychiatry 2014;5:142.

[20] Romli M, Wan Mohamad WN, Awang MA, Aw CL, Zakaria MN. The clinical value of bilateral bone conduction testing in hearing diagnosis. Indian J Otol 2020;26(3):182-5.

[21] Lih AC, Zakaria MN, Mohamad RA, Nor Rashid MF. Effects of ethnicity and gender on the middle ear function in Asian adults. Indian J Otol 2017;23(2):94-7.

[22] Avan P, Giraudet F, Büki B. Importance of binaural hearing. Audiol Neurootol 2015;20 Suppl 1:3-6.

[23] Abdul Wahab NA, Wahab S, Abdul Rahman AH, Sidek D, Zakaria MN. The hyperactivity of efferent auditory system in patients with schizophrenia: a transient evoked otoacoustic emissions study. Psychiatry Investig 2016;13(1):82-8.

[24] Wahab S, Zakaria MN, Sidek D, Abdul Rahman AH, Shah SA, Abdul Wahab NA. Evaluation of auditory hallucinations in patients with schizophrenia: A validation study of the Malay version of Psychotic Symptom Rating Scales (PSYRATS). Psychiatry Res 2015;228(3):462-7.

Chapter 13

Assessing the auditory brainstem function in patients with schizophrenia: An acoustic reflex study

Noor AA Wahab[1], PhD
Suzaily Wahab[2], MMed
Rafidah Mazlan[1], PhD
Mahamad A Awang[3], MClinAud
and Mohd N Zakaria[3], PhD

[1]Audiology Programme, Centre for Rehabilitation & Special Needs Studies, Faculty of Health Sciences, Universiti Kebangsaan Malaysia, Kuala Lumpur, Malaysia
[2]Department of Psychiatry, Faculty of Medicine, Universiti Kebangsaan Malaysia, Jalan Yaacob Latif, Bandar Tun Razak, Cheras, Kuala Lumpur, Malaysia
[3]Audiology Programme, School of Health Sciences, Universiti Sains Malaysia, Kelantan, Malaysia

Abstract

It has been reported that patients with schizophrenia may have problems involving the auditory brainstem. In view of this, it was in our interest to see if acoustic reflex thresholds (ARTs) would be altered in this group of patients. In this case-control study, 27 patients diagnosed with schizophrenia (mean age = 32.3 ± 7.01 years) and 26 healthy controls (mean age = 27.0 ± 4.0 years) were enrolled. The acoustic reflex testing was conducted based on the recommended protocol. Ipsilateral and contralateral ARTs were computed for each patient. As revealed, no significant differences in ARTs were found between the groups in both recording conditions at each of the tested frequencies ($p > 0.05$). To

In: Public Health: Audiology Research in Malaysia
Editors: Mohd N. Zakaria and Joav Merrick
ISBN: 979-8-89530-577-5

conclude, although patients with schizophrenia may have auditory brainstem dysfunctions, it appears that the acoustic reflex test (in both ipsilateral and contralateral conditions) is not particularly useful when assessing those with schizophrenia.

Introduction

Since both peripheral and central auditory pathways are involved in processing auditory inputs, any damage to these regions would result in auditory disorders (1). Those with auditory disorders may complain of symptoms such as hearing difficulties (in quiet and noisy environments) as well as other associated problems (2-5).

In clinical settings, hearing healthcare practitioners will perform several assessments for diagnosing the status of hearing (1, 2, 6-10). Among others, the acoustic reflex test is routinely carried out for the purpose of site of lesion assessment (1, 10, 11). The acoustic reflex is a protective mechanism of the auditory system that involves the contraction of the middle ear muscles in response to loud sounds (10). The contraction of the middle ear muscles helps to dampen the transmission of sound and protect the delicate structures of the inner ear. It can be activated bilaterally (in both ears) or contralaterally (in the opposite ear) when loud sounds are presented (10).

The clinical diagnosis is commonly based on the acoustic reflex threshold (ART), i.e., the minimum intensity of a sound stimulus required to elicit an acoustic reflex response. Normal ARTs are typically between 70 and 100 dB (1). On the other hand, patients who have disruptions or pathologies involving the acoustic reflex pathway may show abnormal ARTs. In particular, those who have problems affecting the middle ear, cochlea, auditory nerve, facial nerve, and superior olivary complex (SOC) would produce elevated ARTs or even an absent acoustic reflex (1, 12).

Delusions, hallucinations, disordered speech and thought patterns, and strange social behaviours are hallmarks of schizophrenia, a complex mental illness (13, 14). Approximately 1% of people worldwide suffer from this complicated and frequently misdiagnosed mental illness (15). Many aspects of schizophrenia have been the subject of extensive research, including its underlying causes, possible treatments, and the influence of environmental factors (15, 16).

It is worth mentioning that in schizophrenic patients, abnormal auditory processing has been shown at both the cortical and subcortical levels (17-19).

In particular, those diagnosed with schizophrenia were found to have abnormal late latency response (LLR) results, implying abnormal auditory processing at the cortical level (17, 18). Meanwhile, abnormal findings in the midbrain region were also documented in schizophrenia patients by means of middle latency response (MLR) testing (19). Additionally, several studies found that the auditory brainstem region could be compromised in patients with schizophrenia (20-24). Advanced assessment methods, including the applications of masking technique and electrophysiological test such as auditory brainstem response (ABR), were used for this purpose. In view of this, it was of interest to see whether the routine audiological test (i.e., acoustic reflex assessment) could be useful in assessing the brainstem function in patients with schizophrenia. As such, the aim of this chapter was to compare ART results (obtained ipsilaterally and contralaterally) between schizophrenic patients and healthy controls.

Our study

In this study that employed a case-control study design, 27 patients with schizophrenia (aged 19-44 years) and 26 healthy volunteers (aged 22-36 years) were recruited. The healthy subjects were randomly selected among medical students and staff members of the University Hospital. Meanwhile, the schizophrenic patients were selected using a purposive sampling method among patients who attended the Psychiatric Clinic, University Hospital.

All of the participants were found to have normal hearing thresholds and normal middle ear function for each ear according to pure tone audiometry and tympanometry assessments (25, 26). The diagnosis of schizophrenia was determined using the DSM-IV and based on Brief Psychotic Rating Scales (BPRS) scores (27), all patients with schizophrenia recruited in the present study were found to be mentally stable and had no severe psychotic conditions.

The acoustic reflex testing was then carried out on each participant based on the recommended protocol (1). To achieve this, the GSI Tympstar middle ear analyzer (Grason-Stadler Inc., USA) was used to determine ipsilateral and contralateral acoustic reflex results. The ipsilateral acoustic reflex assessment was conducted when the probe and the stimulus were positioned in the same ear. On the other hand, in the contralateral acoustic reflex testing, the probe was placed in one ear and the stimulus was presented to the other ear.

For both recording conditions, ARTs were determined using pulsed tones at frequencies of 500 Hz, 1000 Hz, and 2000 Hz. For each participant, the initial intensity level was 75 dB, and the intensity level was increased until the ART was identified. In this regard, the ART was defined as the lowest level of pulsed tone needed to elicit at least a 0.02 mmho deflection in the middle ear admittance.

ARTs elicited by ipsilateral and contralateral stimulations were computed for each participant. As shown by the Shapiro-Wilk test, all data were found to be normally distributed ($p > 0.05$), permitting the use of a parametric statistical test. Particularly, the independent t-test was used to compare ARTs between healthy and schizophrenic groups at all test frequencies for both ipsilateral and contralateral conditions. The statistical outcomes were considered statistically significant when the p values were less than 0.05. The data analysis was performed using the MedCalc software (version 20.006, Ostend, Belgium).

Table 1. Mean and standard deviation (SD) of acoustic reflex threshold at 500 Hz, 1000 Hz and 2000 Hz for each recording condition for healthy control and schizophrenia groups

Recording condition	Frequency (Hz)	Healthy control Mean (SD)	Schizophrenia Mean (SD)	P value
Ipsilateral right	500	87.88 (4.73)	87.96 (5.59)	0.956
	1000	87.69 (5.87)	88.33 (5.19)	0.676
	2000	90.19 (6.40)	90.56 (6.10)	0.830
Ipsilateral left	500	89.42 (6.53)	86.85 (5.91)	0.139
	1000	88.65 (5.40)	88.15 (5.57)	0.742
	2000	91.54 (4.64)	91.11 (5.60)	0.763
Contralateral right	500	94.23 (5.60)	91.48 (6.77)	0.114
	1000	92.31 (5.87)	93.15 (4.63)	0.565
	2000	92.31 (6.96)	94.44 (6.70)	0.262
Contralateral left	500	95.00 (6.00)	92.41 (6.26)	0.131
	1000	94.04 (5.10)	93.70 (4.30)	0.794
	2000	93.85 (6.21)	(5.80)	0.563

Findings

For the healthy group, the mean age was 27.0 ± 4.0 years, and 11 of them were males (of 26 participants). As for the schizophrenic group, the mean age was 32.3 ± 7.0 years with 15 males (of 27 participants).

The comparisons of ART results between the two groups are shown in Table 1. Generally, mean ARTs for both recording conditions across the frequencies were within the normal range (less than 100 dB). As revealed by the t-test, no significant differences in ARTs were noted between the groups in the ipsilateral condition at each of the tested frequencies ($p > 0.05$). A similar pattern was observed in the contralateral condition, i.e., both groups produced comparable ARTs at all tested frequencies ($p > 0.05$).

Discussion

The existing literature provides evidence that abnormal auditory processing could occur not just at the cortical and subcortical regions (17-19), but also at the brainstem level (20-24). Herein, it was suggested that schizophrenic patients may show early signs of sensory dysfunctions, and the ABR test was appropriate to document this (20). In a study by Grillion et al. (20), ABR results were compared between 17 male patients with chronic schizophrenia (mean age = 36.7 ± 7.5 years) and 17 healthy male adults (mean age = 35.3 ± 6.7 years). They found that those with schizophrenia produced ABR waveforms with longer interwave latencies of I-III compared to the healthy controls. In a subsequent study by Igata et al. (21), 30 schizophrenic patients (mean age of 31.8 years) and 20 healthy volunteers (mean age of 29.3 years) underwent the ABR testing with clicks as stimuli (at an intensity level of 80 dBHL). The authors then discovered that at least one of ABR waves (I, II or III) was missing frequently in the schizophrenic group. It was concluded that patients with schizophrenia (particularly those with negative symptoms) may have some auditory processing abnormalities in the lower brainstem (21). In line with this, Källstrand et al. (23) recorded ABR waveforms using the forward masking technique from 5 groups of subjects, i.e., healthy controls (n = 49, mean age of 39.4 years), schizophrenic patients (n = 49, mean age of 41.6 years), attention deficit hyperactivity disorder patients (n = 29, mean age of 36.1 years), Asperger syndrome patients (n = 13, mean age of 38.4 years) and those suffering from drug-induced psychosis (n = 14, mean age of 32.0 years). As reported, abnormal laterality of brainstem activity in the wave II of ABR was seen in the schizophrenic patients (relative to all other study groups), implying deficits in the auditory information coding in the lower parts of the auditory system in schizophrenia. In a more recent study, the ABR testing was found to be highly sensitive (i.e., with a sensitivity value of 84.6%) in detecting brainstem dysfunctions in patients with schizophrenia (24).

In this chapter, the ARTs between the schizophrenic and healthy groups did not differ significantly for both ipsilateral and contralateral recording conditions at all test frequencies. Furthermore, the mean ARTs for the two groups were all within the normal range. In other words, the acoustic reflex test "failed" to identify abnormalities in the auditory pathway in those with schizophrenia. This was rather surprising, as the acoustic reflex test was found to be sensitive in detecting pathologies that occur within the acoustic reflex pathway, including the lower brainstem level (i.e., up to SOC) (1,10-12), which can be compromised in schizophrenic patients.

The inability of the acoustic reflex assessment in detecting possible auditory brainstem problems in patients with schizophrenia could be due to several reasons. First, since the acoustic reflex pathway is only up to the level of SOC (1), it is therefore possible to have normal ARTs if the lesions occur higher than this level. Second, as pointed out by others, auditory assessments that employ more complex stimulations can be more beneficial in identifying brainstem problems in schizophrenia (22,23). In light of this, the routine acoustic reflex test can be considered relatively "simple" and may not be sensitive enough to detect the expected lesions. Lastly, it is also possible that the majority of the schizophrenic patients recruited in the present study may not have auditory brainstem dysfunctions. In line with this, abnormal ABR results could be seen in only a subset of patients with schizophrenia (20). Accordingly, replicating this study using a larger sample size and adding other tests (such as ABR) can be useful to provide further insight into this matter.

The present study's findings, on the other hand, are in line with other reports that revealed normal ABR findings in those with schizophrenia (28-30). In a study by Clayson et al. (30), no significant differences in ABR results were found between patients with schizophrenia (n = 52) and healthy control subjects (n = 32). They then concluded that the brainstem-mediated responses are intact in those with schizophrenia. Owing to the mixed findings in this interesting aspect of schizophrenia, future studies are clearly warranted to provide more credible evidence on the status of auditory processing at the brainstem level in patients suffering from schizophrenia.

Conclusion

Even though patients with schizophrenia may have auditory brainstem dysfunctions, we found no evidence that the routine audiological test, i.e., acoustic reflex assessment, was sensitive enough to identify possible auditory brainstem problems in those patients. Until further evidence emerges, it appears that the acoustic reflex test (in both ipsilateral and contralateral conditions) is not particularly useful when assessing patients with schizophrenia.

Acknowledgments

The authors have stated all possible conflicts of interest within this work. The authors have stated all sources of funding for this work. If this work involved human participants, informed consent was received from each individual. If this work involved human participants, it was conducted in accordance with the 1964 Declaration of Helsinki. If this work involved experiments with humans or animals, it was conducted in accordance with the related institutions' research ethics guidelines.

References

[1] Katz J, Chasin M, English K, Hood L, Tillery KL. Handbook of clinical audiology. Philadelphia, PA: Lippincott Williams Wilkins, 2015.

[2] Wan Mohamad WN, Romli M, Awang MA, Abdullah R, Lih AC, Zakaria MN. The presence of unusual bone conduction thresholds in pure tone audiometry. Indian J Otol 2020;26(1):54-7.

[3] Zainun Z, Zakaria MN, Sidek D, Ismail Z. Clinical use of Malay Version of Vertigo Symptom Scale (MVSS) in patients with peripheral vestibular disorder (PVD). Med J Malaysia 2012;67(4):386-9.

[4] Wong JW, Wan Mohamad WN, Wan Husain WS, Zakaria MN. The tinnitus suppressive effect: Comparisons between three types of maskers. Int J Disabil Hum Dev 2020;19(1):21-6.

[5] Zakaria MN. The effectiveness of sound therapy in treating patients with mild and severe tinnitus. Int J Disabil Hum Dev 2020;19(2):215-9.

[6] Abdul Wahid SN, Md Daud MK, Sidek D, Abd Rahman N, Mansor S, Zakaria MN. The performance of distortion product otoacoustic emissions and automated auditory brainstem response in the same ear of the babies in neonatal unit. Int J Pediatr Otorhinolaryngol 2012;76(9):1366-9.

[7] Jalaei B, Azmi MHAM, Zakaria MN. Gender disparity in binaural speech-evoked auditory brainstem response: are they clinically significant? Braz J Otorhinolaryngol 2019;85:486-93.

[8] Zakaria MN, Jalaei B, Wahab NA. Gender and modulation frequency effects on auditory steady state response (ASSR) thresholds. Eur Arch Otorhinolaryngol 2016;273(2):349-54.

[9] Mukari SZS, Umat C, Chan SC, Ali A, Maamor N, Zakaria MN. Effects of age and type of stimulus on the cortical auditory evoked potential in healthy Malaysian children. J Audiol Otol 2020;24(1):35-9.

[10] Awang MA, Zakaria MN. Acoustic reflex testing in clinical audiology: What is the next direction? Int J Disabil Hum Dev 2019;18(2):123-8.

[11] Awang MA, Zamri NN, Romli M, Zakaria MN. Acoustic reflex latency (ARL) assessment in Malaysian adults: The effects of age, gender and stimulus frequency. NeuroQuantology 2019;17(2):91-6.

[12] Clemis JD. Acoustic reflex testing in otoneurology. Otolaryngol Head Neck Surg 1984;92(2):141-4.

[13] Abdul Wahab NA, Wahab S, Abdul Rahman AH, Sidek D, Zakaria MN. The hyperactivity of efferent auditory system in patients with schizophrenia: a transient evoked otoacoustic emissions study. Psychiatry Investig 2016;13(1):82-8.

[14] Wahab S, Zakaria MN, Sidek D, Abdul Rahman AH, Shah SA, Abdul Wahab NA. Evaluation of auditory hallucinations in patients with schizophrenia: A validation study of the Malay version of Psychotic Symptom Rating Scales (PSYRATS). Psychiatry Res 2015;228(3):462-7.

[15] Kahn RS, Sommer IE, Murray RM, Meyer-Lindenberg A, Weinberger DR, Cannon TD, et al. Schizophrenia. Nat Rev Dis Primers 2015;1:15067.

[16] Gaebel W, Zielasek J. Schizophrenia in 2020: Trends in diagnosis and therapy. Psychiatry Clin Neurosci 2015;69(11):661-73.

[17] Rissling AJ, Miyakoshi M, Sugar CA, Braff DL, Makeig S, Light GA. Cortical substrates and functional correlates of auditory deviance processing deficits in schizophrenia. Neuroimage Clin 2014;6:424-37.

[18] Turetsky BI, Dress EM, Braff DL, Calkins ME, Green MF, Greenwood TA, et al. The utility of P300 as a schizophrenia endophenotype and predictive biomarker: clinical and socio-demographic modulators in COGS-2. Schizophr Res 2015;163(1-3):53-62.

[19] Leavitt VM, Molholm S, Ritter W, Shpaner M, Foxe JJ. Auditory processing in schizophrenia during the middle latency period (10-50 ms): high-density electrical mapping and source analysis reveal subcortical antecedents to early cortical deficits. J Psychiatry Neurosci 2007;32(5):339-53.

[20] Grillon C, Ameli R, Glazer WM. Brainstem auditory-evoked potentials to different rates and intensities of stimulation in schizophrenics. Biol Psychiatry 1990;28(9):819-23.

[21] Igata M, Ohta M, Hayashida Y, Abe K. Missing peaks in auditory brainstem responses and negative symptoms in schizophrenia. Jpn J Psychiatry Neurol 1994;48(3):571-8.

[22] Källstrand J, Montnémery P, Nielzén S, Olsson O. Auditory masking experiments in schizophrenia. Psychiatry Res 2002;113(1-2):115-25.

[23] Källstrand J, Nehlstedt SF, Sköld ML, Nielzén S. Lateral asymmetry and reduced forward masking effect in early brainstem auditory evoked responses in schizophrenia. Psychiatry Res 2012;196(2-3):188-93.

[24] Juselius Baghdassarian E, Nilsson Markhed M, Lindström E, Nilsson BM, Lewander T. Auditory brainstem response (ABR) profiling tests as diagnostic

support for schizophrenia and adult attention-deficit hyperactivity disorder (ADHD). Acta Neuropsychiatr 2018;30(3):137-47.

[25] Lih AC, Zakaria MN, Mohamad RA, Nor Rashid MF. Effects of ethnicity and gender on the middle ear function in Asian adults. Indian J Otol 2017;23(2):94-7.

[26] Romli M, Wan Mohamad WN, Awang MA, Aw CL, Zakaria MN. The clinical value of bilateral bone conduction testing in hearing diagnosis. Indian J Otol 2020;26(3):182-5.

[27] Leucht S, Kane JM, Kissling W, Hamann J, Etschel E, Engel R. Clinical implications of Brief Psychiatric Rating Scale scores. Br J Psychiatry 2005;187:366-71.

[28] McKay CM, Headlam DM, Copolov DL. Central auditory processing in patients with auditory hallucinations. Am J Psychiatry 2000;157(5):759-66.

[29] Nam EC. Is it necessary to differentiate tinnitus from auditory hallucination in schizophrenic patients? J Laryngol Otol 2005;119(5):352-5.

[30] Clayson PE, Joshi YB, Thomas ML, Sprock J, Nungaray J, Swerdlow NR, et al. Click-evoked auditory brainstem responses (ABRs) are intact in schizophrenia and not sensitive to cognitive training. Biomark Neuropsychiatry 2022;6:100046.

Chapter 14

Understanding the neural processing of hearing-impaired children: An aided cortical auditory evoked potential (CAEP) study

Nurnazeha Isnan[1,2], BSc
Rosninda Abdullah[2], MSc
Nik AN Othman[3], MMed
Wan NW Mohamad[2], PhD
Nashrah Maamor[4], PhD
and Mohd N Zakaria[2], PhD

[1]Hospital Putrajaya, Putrajaya, Wilayah Persekutuan Putrajaya, Malaysia
[2]Audiology Programme, School of Health Sciences, Universiti Sains Malaysia, Kelantan, Malaysia
[3]Department of Otorhinolaryngology, School of Medical Sciences, Universiti Sains Malaysia, Kelantan, Malaysia
[4]Centre for Ear, Hearing and Speech, Faculty of Health Sciences, Universiti Kebangsaan Malaysia, Kuala Lumpur, Malaysia

Abstract

Limited studies have investigated the use of cortical auditory evoked potential (CAEP) to measure hearing aid outcomes in children. As such, more research efforts are needed to provide better insight into this aspect. In this chapter, the waveforms of aided CAEP of hearing-impaired children (who used hearing aids consistently) were compared with those of normal children. 18 normal hearing (NH) children and 13 children with sensorineural hearing loss (SNHL) (aged 5 to 12 years) were enrolled in our study. The aided CAEP testing was carried out according

In: Public Health: Audiology Research in Malaysia
Editors: Mohd N. Zakaria and Joav Merrick
ISBN: 979-8-89530-577-5

to the recommended protocol. A natural speech syllable /ba/ was used as the stimulus, and it was presented repetitively at 65 dB SPL using a loudspeaker in a dedicated soundproof room. While sitting comfortably, the children were asked to watch voiceless movies during the CAEP testing. The response rates for each of the CAEP peaks did not differ significantly between the two groups ($p > 0.05$). Except for N_2 amplitude ($p = 0.020$), the amplitudes of other CAEP peaks were not statistically different between NH and SNHL groups ($p > 0.05$). Most of CAEP peaks (N_1, P_2 and N_2) produced latencies that were comparable between the two groups ($p > 0.05$). In contrast, the mean P_1 latency was statistically longer for the SNHL children ($p = 0.018$). To conclude, the SNHL children revealed nearly normal CAEP findings implying the positive outcomes of using hearing aids consistently. Brain maturation appears to continue over time even among hearing aid users. The aided CAEP should be considered as a potential test to document the effectiveness of amplification, particularly among children.

Introduction

Hearing impairment and other auditory symptoms are prevalent health conditions and may greatly reduce the quality of life for those experiencing them (1-5). To accurately identify the extent of hearing difficulties, comprehensive evaluations are essential. In clinical practice, hearing healthcare professionals typically employ a combination of subjective and objective tests to assess the degree and type of hearing loss (6-10). The cortical auditory evoked potential (CAEP), for example, is an objective method for assessing how well the auditory system functions at the cortical level (11, 12).

Following the appropriate hearing diagnosis, the respective patients are treated accordingly. For those diagnosed with conductive hearing loss (CHL), medications and/or surgeries are the typical treatments (11). Hearing amplification devices such as hearing aids and cochlear implants are the common options for improving hearing of individuals with sensorineural hearing loss (SNHL). For optimum outcomes, these hearing amplification devices must be set properly (based on the patient's audiogram) and should be used consistently (11).

The CAEP represents brain responses when stimulated by auditory stimuli, which can be conveniently measured using electrodes placed on the scalp (12, 13). This auditory evoked potential provides information regarding the function of the auditory cortex responsible for processing auditory information. It has several peaks (i.e., P_1, N_1, P_2, and N_2) that have piqued the interest of researchers (11). Studies on CAEP among hearing aid users have been gaining momentum as researchers aim to understand brain processing and flexibility particularly in children (14). However, there are variations in the methodology used in CAEP research, making it necessary to establish a strong knowledge foundation on aided CAEP to improve the current information from this population (15). It is worth stating that CAEP studies in children with hearing impairment are limited, and the feasibility of CAEPs remains unclear clinically (16). The uncertainty in the normative values to be compared with SNHL individuals further highlights the need for research in this area (17).

Recording aided CAEP offers significant advantages in assessing hearing aid fitting in children compared to other electrophysiological test methods (18). By using natural stimuli such as speech sounds, the CAEP can measure how well the sounds are perceived and processed at the cortical area (12, 13). In rare cases such as auditory neuropathy (where the auditory brainstem response (ABR) is absent), the CAEP testing is useful in documenting the aided verification outcomes with the use of hearing aids or cochlear implants (19).

The aided CAEP has the potential to provide valuable information in assessing hearing aid fitting and effectiveness, particularly in children. Establishing a strong knowledge foundation and standardizing the methodology used in the aided CAEP research can help improve the current understanding of this area and inform clinical practice. As such, the aim of this chapter was to investigate whether the CAEP waveforms could be reliably recorded from consistent hearing aid users using the commonly available clinical test equipment. Since the main goal of hearing aid validation procedures is to assess the benefit of hearing aid use while listening to speech, the present study would employ speech stimuli (in the most natural as possible) to evoke CAEP responses.

Our study

In this study that employed a case control research design, eighteen normal hearing (NH) children and thirteen children with SNHL aged 5 to 12 years were enrolled. To ensure their eligibility, all children underwent routine audiological assessments (i.e., otoscopy, pure tone audiometry and tympanometry) based on the recommended protocols (6,10). All of them showed normal tympanograms, implying healthy middle ear function. Based on audiograms, the NH children had hearing within the normal limits (i.e., hearing thresholds $\leq$ 20 dB HL at the tested frequencies), while those with SNHL had hearing loss ranging from mild to severe degree of loss. Prior to the CAEP assessment, the hearing aids of children with SNHL underwent verification to ensure the behavioural outputs were within the speech spectrum (at children's preferred settings).

A two-channel Biologic Navigator Pro AEP device (Natus Medical Inc., Mundelein, USA) was used in the CAEP testing. In terms of the placement of electrodes, the inverting electrode was placed at the top middle of the head (Cz), the non-inverting electrode at the mastoid (contralateral to the hand dominance), and the common electrode at the high forehead (Fpz). The impedance of each electrode was maintained below 5 kΩ during the testing. Stimuli to be used were constructed from running speech spoken by a middle-aged female whose native language is Malay language. The speech syllable /ba/ (duration of 70 ms) was identified and extracted within the soundtrack that was recorded in the soundproof room using a Sennheiser microphone.

The CAEP testing was carried out according to the recommended protocol for both groups. The testing was conducted in binaural listening condition for the NH group and in binaural-aided condition for the SNHL group (using bilateral hearing aids). At a stimulus rate of 1.1/s, the speech syllable /ba/ was presented at an intensity of 65 dB SPL through a loudspeaker. While sitting comfortably, the children were asked to watch voiceless movies during the testing. The recording was repeated to corroborate replicability between the first and second recordings. The filter setting was set at 1-30 Hz and at least 150 sweeps were obtained for each trial.

Two experts in the field of auditory electrophysiology were involved in confirming the peaks of CAEP. The response rates, latencies and amplitudes of P_1, N_1, P_2 and N_2 for each child were then documented. The Shapiro-Wilk test was used to determine the data distribution. Since the data were found to be normally distributed ($p > 0.05$), the appropriate parametric statistical test was conducted as applicable. In particular, the independent t-test was employed to compare CAEP amplitudes and latencies between NH and SNHL groups. For comparing the response rates between the two groups, the chi-square analysis was employed. The p value of less than 0.05 was considered statistically significant. The MedCalc software (version 20.006, Ostend, Belgium) was used in the data analysis.

Findings

The mean age of children who participated in the present study was 7.89 ± 2.03 years. They were all Malay, with a balanced gender distribution for each group. The response rates for each of the CAEP peaks for NH and SNHL groups are shown in Figure 1. As illustrated, for both groups, the response rates for P_1 and N_1 peaks were 100%. The response rates were slightly lower for P_2 and N_2 peaks. As revealed in the chi-square analysis, the response rates for all CAEP peaks did not differ significantly between the two groups ($p > 0.05$).

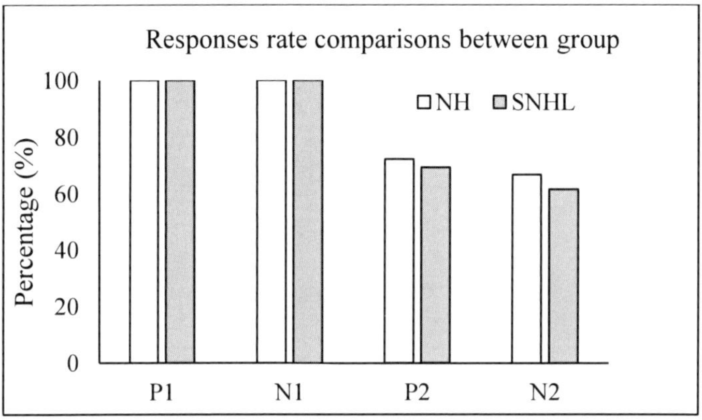

Figure 1. The response rate of each peak of cortical auditory evoked potential (CAEP) for normal hearing (NH) and sensorineural hearing loss (SNHL) groups.

The statistical outcomes when the CAEP amplitudes were compared between NH and SNHL children are shown in Table 1. Descriptively, the mean amplitudes for all CAEP peaks were found to be higher for the NH group. As indicated in the t-test analysis, except for N_2 amplitude, all CAEP amplitudes were found to be comparable between the two groups ($p > 0.05$). On the other hand, the mean N_2 amplitude produced by the NH group was statistically higher than that of the SNHL group ($p = 0.020$).

Table 2 shows the statistical results when the CAEP latencies were compared between NH and SNHL groups. It can be seen that for all CAEP peaks, the SNHL children produced descriptively longer mean latencies. This observation was supported by the t-test analysis, i.e., the mean P_1 latency was statistically longer in the SNHL group than in the NH group ($p = 0.018$).

Nevertheless, other CAEP peaks (N_1, P_2 and N_2) produced mean latencies that did not differ significantly between the two groups ($p > 0.05$) (Table 2).

Table 1. Statistical results when cortical auditory evoked potential (CAEP) amplitudes are compared between normal hearing (NH) and sensorineural hearing loss (SNHL) children

Amplitude (μV)	NH Mean (SD)	SNHL Mean (SD)	P value
P1	4.18 (1.55)	3.32 (1.25)	0.110
N1	6.82 (3.57)	4.82 (2.24)	0.086
P2	2.95(1.78)	2.18 (1.19)	0.186
N2	3.02 (2.37)	1.33 (0.78)	*0.020

*Significant at $p < 0.05$.

Table 2. Statistical results when cortical auditory evoked potential (CAEP) latencies are compared between normal hearing (NH) and sensorineural hearing loss (SNHL) children

Latency (ms)	NH Mean (SD)	SNHL Mean (SD)	P value
P1	111.74 (27.66)	140.94 (36.98)	*0.018
N1	216.01 (51.18)	242.72 (35.96)	0.118
P2	339.93 (96.86)	370.09 (45.26)	0.307
N2	392.99 (79.07)	441.05 (36.79)	0.052

*Significant at $p < 0.05$.

Discussion

The present study aimed to compare the waveforms of aided CAEP of hearing-impaired children with those of normal-hearing children. The results of this study suggest that the SNHL children revealed nearly normal CAEP findings, implying the positive outcomes of using hearing aids consistently (20, 21). The development of brain maturation appears to continue over time even among hearing aid users. The findings of this study are in line with those of previous studies demonstrating that the use of hearing aids can lead to improvements in CAEP responses in children with SNHL (22, 23).

Interestingly, the response rates for each of CAEP peaks did not differ significantly between the NH and SNHL groups. This suggests that the use of hearing aids may help restore the neural responses to auditory stimuli in children with SNHL to levels similar to those observed in the NH children. The fact that the amplitudes and latencies of most CAEP peaks were comparable between the two groups further supports this idea. However, the P_1 latency and N_2 amplitude were found to be statistically different between the NH and SNHL children. This implies that there may be some differences in the neural processing of auditory stimuli between NH and SNHL children, even when the SNHL children use hearing aids. Perhaps the use of hearing aids consistently for a longer duration would improve these CAEP peaks, and this is subject to further research.

The present study has some limitations that should be considered when interpreting the results. Firstly, the sample size used was relatively small, which may limit the generalizability of the findings. Future studies with larger sample sizes are needed to verify the findings of the present study. Secondly, this study only examined the short-term effects of hearing aid use on CAEP responses. Longitudinal studies are needed to investigate the long-term effects of hearing aid use on CAEP responses in children with SNHL. Finally, the study only assessed the effects of hearing aid use on CAEP responses to a single speech syllable. Future studies should investigate the effects of hearing aid use on CAEP waveforms when stimulated by different types of speech stimuli.

Despite these limitations, the present study provides important insights into the use of CAEP as a potential test to document the effectiveness of amplification, particularly among children. The findings of this study suggest that the CAEP assessment can be used conveniently to evaluate the outcomes of hearing aid use in children with SNHL. As reported elsewhere, CAEP is an objective measure that is not affected by factors such as attention, motivation, and language development, which are known to affect the results of behavioural tests.

Conclusion

In conclusion, the present study compared CAEP results between NH children and children with SNHL who used hearing aids consistently. The findings revealed comparable response rates between the groups, with no significant differences in amplitudes or latencies for most of the CAEP peaks. Overall, the SNHL group demonstrated near-normal CAEP responses, suggesting that the hearing aid use helped restore neural processing of auditory information to levels approximating NH peers. While longitudinal research on the long-term amplification effects is warranted along with testing using additional stimuli, these preliminary results support the feasibility and potential utility of aided CAEP testing to verify and document benefits from paediatric hearing aid fitting. This objective electrophysiological approach complements existing subjective behavioural measures for validating functional auditory outcomes in children with hearing loss.

Acknowledgments

The authors are thankful to the children and families who participated in this study. This study was funded by a research grant registered under Universiti Sains Malaysia with Project Code: 304/PPSK/6150273.

The authors have stated all possible conflicts of interest within this work. The authors have stated all sources of funding for this work. If this work involved human participants, informed consent was received from each individual. If this work involved human participants, it was conducted in accordance with the 1964 Declaration of Helsinki. If this work involved experiments with humans or animals, it was conducted in accordance with the related institutions' research ethics guidelines.

References

[1] Zuraida Z, Mohd Normani Z, Dinsuhaimi S, Zalina I, Geshina MS. Development of Malay version of vertigo symptom scale (MVVSS) for clinical use. Malaysian J Med Health Sci 2010;6(2):31-9.

[2] Romli M, Wan Mohamad WN, Awang MA, Aw CL, Zakaria MN. The clinical value of bilateral bone conduction testing in hearing diagnosis. Indian J Otol 2020;26(3):182-5.

[3] Wong JW, Wan Mohamad WN, Wan Husain WS, Zakaria MN. The tinnitus suppressive effect: Comparisons between three types of maskers. Int J Disabil Hum Dev 2020;19(1):21-6.

[4] Zakaria MN. The effectiveness of sound therapy in treating patients with mild and severe tinnitus. Int J Disabil Hum Dev 2020;19(2):215-9.

[5] Wahab S, Zakaria MN, Sidek D, Abdul Rahman AH, Shah SA, Abdul Wahab NA. Evaluation of auditory hallucinations in patients with schizophrenia: A validation study of the Malay version of Psychotic Symptom Rating Scales (PSYRATS). Psychiatry Res 2015;228(3):462-7.

[6] Wan Mohamad WN, Romli M, Awang MA, Abdullah R, Lih AC, Zakaria MN. The presence of unusual bone conduction thresholds in pure tone audiometry. Indian J Otol 2020;26(1):54-7.
[7] Abdul Wahid SN, Md Daud MK, Sidek D, Abd Rahman N, Mansor S, Zakaria MN. The performance of distortion product otoacoustic emissions and automated auditory brainstem response in the same ear of the babies in neonatal unit. Int J Pediatr Otorhinolaryngol 2012;76(9):1366-9.
[8] Jalaei B, Azmi MHAM, Zakaria MN. Gender differences in binaural speech-evoked auditory brainstem response: are they clinically significant? Braz J Otorhinolaryngol 2019;85(4):486-93.
[9] Abdul Wahab NA, Wahab S, Abdul Rahman AH, Sidek D, Zakaria MN. The hyperactivity of efferent auditory system in patients with schizophrenia: a transient evoked otoacoustic emissions study. Psychiatry Investig 2016;13(1):82-8.
[10] Lih AC, Zakaria MN, Mohamad RA, Nor Rashid MF. Effects of ethnicity and gender on the middle ear function in Asian adults. Indian J Otol 2017;23(2):94-7.
[11] Katz J, Marshall C, English K, Hood L, Tillery KL. Handbook of clinical audiology. Philadelphia: Lippincott Williams & Wilkins, 2015.
[12] Mukari SZS, Umat C, Chan SC, Ali A, Maamor N, Zakaria MN. Effects of age and type of stimulus on the cortical auditory evoked potential in healthy Malaysian children. J Audiol Otol 2020;24(1):35-9.
[13] Hall JW. New handbook of auditory evoked responses. Boston, MA: Pearson, 2007.
[14] Soleimani M, Rouhbakhsh N, Rahbar N. Towards early intervention of hearing instruments using cortical auditory evoked potentials (CAEPs): A systematic review. Int J Pediatr Otorhinolaryngol 2021;144:110698.
[15] Cone-Wesson B, Wunderlich J. Auditory evoked potentials from the cortex: audiology applications. Curr Opin Otolaryngol Head Neck Surg 2003;11(5):372-7.
[16] Souza PE, Tremblay KL. New perspectives on assessing amplification effects. Trends Amplif 2006;10(3):119-43.
[17] Wunderlich JL, Cone-Wesson BK, Shepherd R. Maturation of the cortical auditory evoked potential in infants and young children. Hear Res 2006;212(1-2):185-202.
[18] Mehta K, Watkin P, Baldwin M, Marriage J, Mahon M, Vickers D. Role of cortical auditory evoked potentials in reducing the age at hearing aid fitting in children with hearing loss identified by newborn hearing screening. Trends Hear 2017;21:2331216517744094.
[19] Punch S, Van Dun B, King A, Carter L, Pearce W. Clinical experience of using cortical auditory evoked potentials in the treatment of infant hearing loss in Australia. Semin Hear 2016;37(1):36-52.
[20] Tomblin JB, Harrison M, Ambrose SE, Walker EA, Oleson JJ, Moeller MP. Language outcomes in young children with mild to severe hearing loss. Ear Hear 2015;36 Suppl 1:76S-91S.
[21] Gabr TA, Kotait MA. Cochlear implant versus hearing aids: cortical auditory-evoked potentials study. Hear Balance Commun 2018;16(1):56-63.
[22] Hazzaa N, Hassan DM, Hassan A. Evaluation of non-linear frequency compression hearing aids using speech P1-cortical auditory evoked potential. Hear Balance Commun 2016;14(1):36-43.

[23] Nash-Kille A, Sharma A. Inter-trial coherence as a marker of cortical phase synchrony in children with sensorineural hearing loss and auditory neuropathy spectrum disorder fitted with hearing aids and cochlear implants. Clin Neurophysiol 2014;125(7):1459-70.

Section three: Miscellaneous issues

Chapter 15

Pure tone audiometry (PTA) and cross-hearing

Mohd N Zakaria[1], PhD
Nik AN Othman[2], MMed
Cheu L Aw[1], MClinAud
Mohd FN Rashid[1], PhD
Mahamad A Awang[1], MClinAud
Wan NW Mohamad[1], PhD
and Rafidah Mazlan[3], PhD

[1]Audiology Programme, School of Health Sciences, Universiti Sains Malaysia, Kelantan, Malaysia
[2]Department of Otorhinolaryngology, School of Medical Sciences, Universiti Sains Malaysia, Kelantan, Malaysia
[3]Audiology Programme, Center for Rehabilitation and Special Needs Studies, Faculty of Health Sciences, Universiti Kebangsaan Malaysia, Kuala Lumpur, Malaysia

Abstract

In pure tone audiometry (PTA) testing, cross-hearing may occur that necessitates the use of masking so that valid air conduction (AC) and bone conduction (BC) thresholds can be obtained. Among others, the presence of a shadow curve on the audiogram has been regarded as an important indicator that the cross-hearing has occurred. In this chapter, we report two cases demonstrating the presence of the shadow curve in PTA even though there is no evidence of cross-hearing. This information can be useful to provide hearing healthcare professionals when dealing with masking cases in PTA.

In: Public Health: Audiology Research in Malaysia
Editors: Mohd N. Zakaria and Joav Merrick
ISBN: 979-8-89530-577-5

Introduction

Hearing loss and related auditory disorders are reasonably common in adults and children (1-5). As such, it is imperative to perform comprehensive hearing assessments (that consist of objective and subjective tests) to achieve accurate hearing diagnoses in clinical settings (6-9). Pure tone audiometry (PTA) has been regarded as the gold standard test for hearing diagnosis (1, 6, 7). Plotted on an audiogram, air conduction (AC) and bone conduction (BC) thresholds are useful to provide information on the severity of hearing loss and the type of hearing loss, respectively (1).

In the AC testing, transducers (such as headphones) are placed comfortably on each ear and used to deliver the respective pure tones. Nevertheless, it is worth stating that the transducers tend to vibrate when presenting auditory stimuli at moderate to high intensity levels, which in turn stimulates the bone conduction pathway (6). In unilateral or asymmetrical hearing loss cases, cross-hearing would occur, and the result obtained from the ear being tested (i.e., the worse ear) would be invalid. The occurrence of cross-hearing is supported by the presence of a shadow curve in the worse ear on the audiogram (i.e., the pattern of AC thresholds for the worse ear is similar to the pattern of AC thresholds for the better ear but with different severity) (10, 11). To avoid cross-hearing (by the non-test ear), a masking procedure is typically carried out and the exact AC thresholds are then determined accordingly (6).

When shadow curves are noted on audiograms, it is likely that the cross-hearing has occurred, and the respective masking procedure should be performed to obtain valid AC thresholds. Additionally, the presence of the shadow curve is considered as an essential indicator for differentiating those with non-organic hearing loss (10). Nevertheless, given the variabilities of otological cases seen in clinical settings, it is also possible that the shadow curve may appear circumstantially. In this paper, we report two rare cases to highlight that the shadow curve on audiograms could occur even though there is no evidence of cross-hearing.

Case report 1

The first case (patient A) was a 64-year-old Malay man who was referred from the Otorhinolaryngology (ORL) Clinic for audiological assessments. His main complaint was disturbing tinnitus in his right ear that occurred about a year ago. The tinnitus was described as continuous, high-pitch, and its loudness increased over time. He also noticed that he had some difficulty hearing when someone was talking, especially in the presence of background noise. He felt that his hearing in the right ear was worse than in the left ear. No complaints of otalgia, otorrhea and vertigo were reported. He was generally healthy and had no other medical illnesses.

During his visit to the Audiology Clinic, University Hospital, the otoscopic examination revealed unremarkable findings. That is, his tympanic membranes were found to be intact with clear ear canals bilaterally. To assess his middle ear function, a 226-Hz tympanometer (AT235H, Interacoustics, Denmark) was utilized. As found, a type A tympanogram was obtained for each ear, indicating a healthy middle ear function. In line with this, his acoustic reflex thresholds (ARTs) were found to be within the normal limits at 500 Hz, 1000 Hz and 2000 Hz (85-100 dB), when tested ipsilaterally and contralaterally. The PTA testing was carried out using a two-channel audiometer (GSI 61, Grason-Stadler Inc, United States) with the respective transducers (TDH-39 headphones and B-71 bone vibrator). Figure 1 shows the PTA result of patient A. As illustrated, he was found to have a mild sensorineural hearing loss (SNHL) in his left ear. In the right ear, a mild to moderate SNHL was noted. Interestingly, the pattern of AC thresholds for the right ear was "strangely" similar to the shape of AC thresholds for the left ear (i.e., the presence of a shadow curve). Nevertheless, differences between left and right AC thresholds were below the minimum suggested value for the need of masking (i.e., 40 dB),[1] indicating that cross-hearing may not occur. Anyway, an AC masking procedure was conducted (with a narrow-band noise presented to the left ear) at all tested frequencies. As expected, the masked AC thresholds were unchanged (compared to those of the unmasked), ascertaining that the cross-hearing did not happen and that the shadow curve was present by chance. It is worth noting that all devices were calibrated and functioning well. In addition, patient A was also asked to rate his tinnitus loudness and annoyance caused by the tinnitus using the respective 10-point visual analogue scale (VAS). For VAS of tinnitus loudness, 0 denotes "not audible" and 10 represents "extremely loud." While for VAS of tinnitus annoyance, 0 represents “not annoying,” while 10 corresponds to “extremely annoying.” He rated her tinnitus loudness and tinnitus annoyance as 7 and 5, respectively.

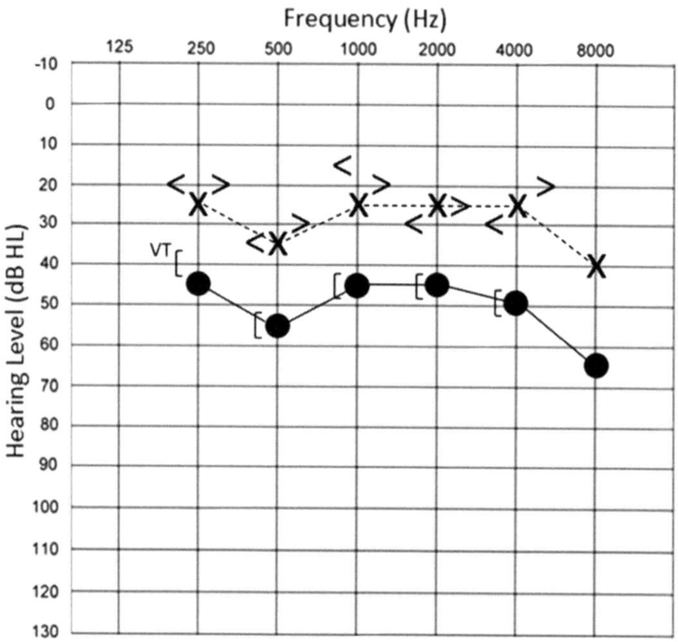

Figure 1. Pure tone audiometry (PTA) result of patient A.

Case report 2

The second case (patient B) was about a 27-year-old Malay female who visited the Audiology Clinic, University Hospital, with the main complaint of reduced hearing in the right ear since childhood. She felt that her hearing became worse gradually over time. Most of the time, she used her left ear (which was claimed to be good) to understand communications and during phone conversations. Her hearing problems were more prominent in the presence of background noise. She was also unable to localize sounds correctly and felt “unsafe” in busy environments. She reported to have intermittent high-pitched tinnitus (but did not disturb her daily life). No history of otalgia, otorrhea, vertigo or other problems related to the ear, nose, or throat was reported.

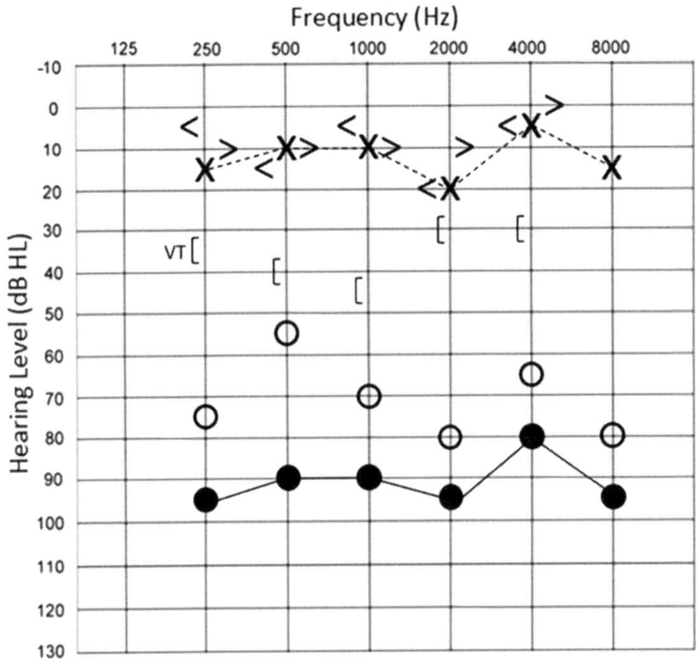

Figure 2. Pure tone audiometry (PTA) result of patient B.

Patient B was found to have an intact tympanic membrane with a clear canal for the left ear, as shown in the otoscopic examination. On the other hand, while having a clear auditory canal, her right tympanic membrane looked dull. In the tympanometric testing, a type A tympanogram (with a compliance value of 0.32 ml) was obtained for the right ear (implying a normal middle ear function). In contrast, a type A_D tympanogram (with a compliance value of 2.07 ml) was noted for her left ear (indicative of hypermobility of tympanic membrane). Due to the high compliance value, no acoustic reflex responses were observed at 500 Hz, 1000 Hz and 2000 Hz when the probe was placed in the left ear (ipsilaterally and contralaterally). Absent acoustic reflexes were also noted in ipsilateral and contralateral conditions for the right ear. The PTA result of patient B is illustrated in Figure 2. As clearly shown, her hearing was found to be within the normal limits in the left ear. Due to notable differences in unmasked AC thresholds between the left and right ears (> 40 dB) and cross-hearing may occur, the AC masking procedure was performed to obtain exact (masked) AC thresholds for the right ear. The masking procedure was indeed successful, and masked AC thresholds were obtained at all tested frequencies (see Figure 2). Based on this information, he was found to have a severe to profound mixed hearing loss in the right ear. Surprisingly, a shadow pattern was noted (see figure 2), in which the shape of masked AC thresholds for the right ear was identical to the pattern of AC thresholds for the left ear.

Discussion

In the PTA testing, when sounds presented to the test ear are loud enough to cause headphones vibrate, they are able to cross-over and be heard by the opposite (non-test) ear through the bone conduction mechanism (1, 12). As such, an appropriate masking procedure must be carried out to deal with the cross-hearing phenomenon so that accurate hearing thresholds can be obtained. However, an interaural attenuation (IAA) process will take place, in which the sound energy will be absorbed by the skull. Herein, in order for cross-hearing to occur, sensibly the sound level should exceed the IAA value (12). The reported IAA values from the previous studies ranged from 35-85 dB (13, 14). In clinical practice, the minimum IAA value of 40 dB has been used to justify the requirement for masking with headphones as the transducers (1, 12).

As demonstrated, the audiogram for patient A revealed the presence of the shadow curve in the right ear. As shown in Figure 1, the differences in AC thresholds between left and right ears ranged from 20-25 dB. On the other hand, the differences between AC thresholds of the right ear and BC thresholds of the left ear were in a range of 20-30 dB. These values were lower than those reported in the literature (12-14). On another note, it is also possible to observe a genuine AC threshold shift (after the masking procedure) even though the IAA value was around 30 dB (12). In view of this, the masking procedure was still carried out accordingly, and the right AC thresholds remained unchanged. This implies that the cross-hearing did not occur and that the presence of the shadow curve on the audiogram was merely circumstantial.

As for patient B, the shadow curve on the audiogram was noted after the masking procedure for the right ear (see Figure 2). Based on the established rules of masking (1, 12), the right AC masking (i.e., the masking noise presented to the left ear) was clearly required at all tested frequencies. In fact, upon the completion of the masking procedure for the right ear, significant AC threshold shifts were observed (up to 35 dB) (see Figure 2). In this regard, when the unmasked right AC thresholds were measured, the cross-hearing phenomenon had occurred, and the tones were subsequently heard by the left (non-test) ear. By performing the essential masking procedure, the exact AC thresholds were able to be documented (to achieve an accurate severity of hearing loss). Interestingly, the shape of masked right AC thresholds was "coincidentally" identical to the shape of left AC thresholds. Taken together, for patient B, it is clear that the presence of the shadow curve on the audiogram had no relation with the cross-hearing phenomenon (as a complete masking procedure had been carefully carried out), and that it happened by chance.

The tympanometric results of patient B are worthy of a further consideration. Since her hearing was within the normal limits in the left ear (with no significant air-bone gaps) (see Figure 2), the "abnormally" high middle ear compliance (as indicated by the type A_D tympanogram) may not indicate the presence of a conductive pathology. It is worth stating that the clinically used normative data on tympanometric parameters (e.g., 0.3-1.6 ml for middle ear compliance) were derived from the study findings involving only 90% of healthy subjects (15-17). In this regard, it seems possible that some individuals with higher compliance values in fact have healthy middle ears (as supported by other test results including those of PTA). If this assumption was true for patient B, the "normal" tympanogram obtained for her right ear (with the compliance value of 0.32 ml) might indicate the presence of the conductive pathology. That is, if she was "born" with "abnormally" high middle ear compliance in both ears, the decreased compliance value in the right ear could be considered "abnormal". Furthermore, if this possibility is agreeable, the tympanometric finding for the right ear is now consistent with the significant air-bone gaps seen in Figure 2.

In terms of case management, patient A was scheduled to undergo the site of lesion assessments (i.e., tone decay, reflex decay, and auditory brainstem response) in his next appointment to rule out the presence of acoustic neuroma. He was also referred to a specialized tinnitus clinic to assess and manage his disturbing tinnitus. While for patient B, she was referred to an ORL specialist to treat the possible conductive pathology (that contributed to mixed type of hearing loss in her right ear) and she will be seen again after the medical management.

Conclusion

In clinical settings, PTA results are important to have complete hearing diagnoses. As applicable, the masking procedure must be implemented since cross-hearing may occur during the PTA testing. Among others, the presence of the shadow curve on the audiogram has been regarded as an important indicator that the cross-hearing has occurred. Nevertheless, as reported in this paper, the shadow curve in PTA may appear even though there is no evidence of cross-hearing. As such, the established rules for masking should be the main indicator that the cross-hearing has occurred (rather than the presence of the shadow curve).

Declaration of patient consent

The authors certify that they have obtained the consent form from the patients. In the form, the patients have given their consent for their image and other clinical information to be reported in the journal. The patients understand that their name and initial will not be published, and due efforts will be made to conceal their identity, but anonymity cannot be guaranteed.

References

[1] Katz J, Marshall C, English K, Hood L, Tillery KL. Handbook of clinical audiology. Philadelphia, PA: Lippincott Williams Wilkins, 2015.

[2] Zuraida Z, Mohd Normani Z, Dinsuhaimi S, Zalina I, Geshina MS. Development of Malay version of vertigo symptom scale (MVVSS) for clinical use. Malaysian J Med Health Sci 2010;6(2):31-9.

[3] Wong JW, Wan Mohamad WN, Wan Husain WS, Zakaria MN. The tinnitus suppressive effect: Comparisons between three types of maskers. Int J Disabil Hum Dev 2020;19(1):21-6.

[4] Zakaria MN. The effectiveness of sound therapy in treating patients with mild and severe tinnitus. Int J Disabil Hum Dev 2020;19(2):215-9.

[5] Wahab S, Zakaria MN, Sidek D, Abdul Rahman AH, Shah SA, Abdul Wahab NA. Evaluation of auditory hallucinations in patients with schizophrenia: A validation study of the Malay version of Psychotic Symptom Rating Scales (PSYRATS). Psychiatry Res 2015;228(3):462-7.

[6] Wan Mohamad WN, Romli M, Awang MA, Abdullah R, Lih AC, Zakaria MN. The presence of unusual bone conduction thresholds in pure tone audiometry. Indian J Otol 2020;26(1):54-7.

[7] Romli M, Wan Mohamad WN, Awang MA, Aw CL, Zakaria MN. The clinical value of bilateral bone conduction testing in hearing diagnosis. Indian J Otol 2020;26(3):182-5.

[8] Jalaei B, Azmi MHAM, Zakaria MN. Gender differences in binaural speech-evoked auditory brainstem response: are they clinically significant? Braz J Otorhinolaryngol 2019;85(4):486-93.

[9] Abdul Wahab NA, Wahab S, Abdul Rahman AH, Sidek D, Zakaria MN. The hyperactivity of efferent auditory system in patients with schizophrenia: a transient evoked otoacoustic emissions study. Psychiatry Investig 2016;13(1):82-8.

[10] Jerger S, Jerger J. Functional hearing disorders: Auditory disorders. Boston, MA: College Hill Press, 1981.

[11] Tschiassny K. Mechanism of shadow hearing. AMA Arch Otolaryngol 1952;55(1):22-30.

[12] Zakaria MN. The importance of considering the minimum interaural attenuation value in the masking procedure of pure-tone audiometry. Indian J Otol 2022;28(2):153-5.

[13] Bunch CC. Auditory tests in cases of complete unilateral deafness. Ann Otol Rhinol Laryngol 1931;40:748-62.

[14] Park YJ, Park KH, Jun GE, Oh SK, Lee CK. Evaluation of the interaural attenuation for pure tone audiometry in Korean. Korean J Audiol 2011;15(1):32-6.

[15] Shahnaz N, Davies D. Standard and multifrequency tympanometric norms for Caucasian and Chinese young adults. Ear Hear 2006;27(1):75-90.

[16] Wahab NA, Rashid MF. Tympanometric values in young Malay adults: preliminary data. Singapore Med J 2009;50(11):1077-9.

[17] Lih AC, Zakaria MN, Mohamad RA, Nor Rashid MF. Effects of ethnicity and gender on the middle ear function in Asian adults. Indian J Otol 2017;23(2):94-7.

Chapter 16

The effect of electrode montage on the aided cortical auditory evoked potential (CAEP)

Nurnazeha Isnan[1,2], BSc
Rosninda Abdullah[2], MSc
Nik AN Othman[3], MMed
Wan NW Mohamad[2], PhD
Nashrah Maamor[4], PhD
and Mohd N Zakaria[2], PhD

[1]Putrajaya Hospital, Putrajaya, Wilayah Persekutuan Putrajaya, Malaysia
[2]Audiology Programme, School of Health Sciences, Universiti Sains Malaysia, Kelantan, Malaysia
[3]Department of Otorhinolaryngology, School of Medical Sciences, Universiti Sains Malaysia, Kelantan, Malaysia
[4] Centre for Ear, Hearing and Speech, Faculty of Health Sciences, Universiti Kebangsaan Malaysia, Kuala Lumpur, Malaysia

Abstract

Cortical auditory evoked potential (CAEP) can be used to assess the auditory pathway function in hearing aid users, but the optimal protocol remains unclear. This chapter examined the influence of electrode montage on CAEP in an aided child with hearing impairment. A 10-year-old girl with moderate sensorineural hearing loss bilaterally (and were fitted with hearing aids at five years of age) underwent the aided CAEP testing using two electrode positions: T_3 and vertex (Cz). Four speech stimuli (/ba/, /m/, /g/, and /t/) were presented to record CAEP waveforms. While both electrode positions revealed robust P1-N1-P2 and N2 responses, the Cz position revealed CAEP waveforms with better

In: Public Health: Audiology Research in Malaysia
Editors: Mohd N. Zakaria and Joav Merrick
ISBN: 979-8-89530-577-5

morphology. Furthermore, relative to the T_3 position, the majority of CAEP peaks showed higher amplitudes for the Cz position. On the other hand, the latencies of most CAEP peaks were descriptively shorter for the T_3 position. Collectively, the study findings suggest that the multi-electrode recording of CAEP would be the best approach in determining the intervention benefits; the Cz position confirms audibility, while the T_3 position represents speech-language development. Tailoring the electrode montage of CAEP to differentiate sensory and cognitive processes provides a greater insight into the auditory status beyond audibility alone. The standard CAEP protocols should include midline and lateral electrodes to distinguish basic improvements from higher cognitive functions in guiding targeted rehabilitation needs.

Introduction

Having good hearing is essential for carrying out daily tasks. The occurrence of hearing loss and related auditory problems may significantly impair the quality of life of the affected individuals (1-5). Thorough hearing assessments are therefore needed to properly diagnose the hearing status. In clinical settings, both subjective and objective hearing assessments are conducted to determine the severity of hearing loss, as well as the type of hearing loss (6-8). Among other tests, the cortical auditory evoked potential (CAEP) is an objective tool for assessing how well the auditory system functions at the cortical levels (8-10).

The CAEP has many potential applications, but it is also useful for quantifying the improvement achieved by using hearing aids in hearing loss cases (11-13). This electrophysiological test is therefore advantageous to provide objective information regarding the benefits of hearing aids in children and complex paediatric cases. However, the CAEP results may vary depending on the type of stimulus and recording parameters (9, 12, 14). This potential variability is still unclear, depending on individual and research experiments (12).

Despite the fact that the CAEP waveform has four peaks, the first prominent peak (P_1) is commonly highlighted in the literature as it has been identified as a reliable biomarker. Other CAEP peaks, such as N_1, P_2, and N_2, are less commonly reported in children due to their greater variability. Having specific normative data is essential so that the CAEP assessment can be used conveniently for its intended applications (15). Nevertheless, this electrophysiological test is not widely used in clinical practice for a variety of reasons, including a lack of expert availability to record CAEP. Furthermore, variations in stimulus and recording parameters (such as different electrode montages) may affect the CAEP waveforms (14). In view of this, little is known regarding which electrode placement is preferred for recording aided CAEP responses from those with hearing impairment. In this paper, the influence of electrode montage on CAEP peaks was studied in a hearing-impaired child who used hearing aids consistently.

Case report

This is the case of a 10-year-old Malay girl who was referred from a district clinic because her speech was unintelligible to others. According to the case history, the child was born full-term via spontaneous vaginal delivery (SVD), weighing 3.40 kg. The antenatal and neonatal history were uneventful. In terms of physical development, she could sit at nine months and began walking around the age of one year. She was hospitalized for vital sign monitoring following a drowning incident last year. Given her brother's diagnosis of sensorineural hearing loss (SNHL) and the use of hearing aids, she has a strong family history of deafness. She also has cousins fitted with cochlear implants. She is the fifth sibling out of seven in the family.

When the child was five years old, her mother took her to the Audiology Clinic, University Hospital for hearing evaluations. The otoscopic examination conducted on the initial visit demonstrated a normal view of the tympanic membrane and ear canal for each ear. Type A tympanograms were obtained from the tympanometry, which suggested healthy middle ears. The distortion product otoacoustic emission (DPOAE) test showed bilateral "refer" results at all tested frequencies (1.5 kHz to 5 kHz), indicating poor outer hair cell emissions. The play audiometry was performed with insert earphones; however, because of her uncooperativeness, the results were incomplete. Subsequently, the free-field testing revealed moderate to severe hearing loss, at least in the better ear.

The girl and her mother returned the following month for the second visit to complete the hearing assessment. During this visit, the child was diagnosed with moderate hearing loss bilaterally with play audiometry. However, the bone conduction testing was not performed due to the child's lack of attention. The child was advised to wear hearing aids to improve her hearing and speech abilities.

In the subsequent visit, the child was reported to use hearing aids three months after being diagnosed and receive welfare funding for them. Her mother stated that her daughter responded well to hearing aids, which significantly improved her speech pronunciation and preparedness for school (as the child will start school at 7 years of age). In order to monitor her hearing and speech skills, the girl has been seeing a speech therapist and an audiologist on a regular basis. She also wears her hearing aids for five to seven hours a day on average. She currently attends a typical school and performs academically on par.

The CAEP testing was then carried out using a modified protocol and Biologic Navigator Pro AEP device. Natural speech stimuli (speech syllable: /ba/ and speech phonemes: /m/, /g/, and /t/) were delivered at a rate of 1.1/s using a loudspeaker at 65 dB SPL. The testing was held in a sound-proofed room, with the child occupied with a puzzle-solving game to keep her awake. The electrodes were placed hemispherically, i.e., inverting electrodes at T_3 and Cz locations and a non-inverting electrode at the mastoid (M1), with the high forehead (Fpz) serving as a common electrode (Figure 1). The impedance of electrodes was kept below 5 kΩ throughout the testing. The child hemispheric dominance was ascertained by her writing hand (right hand). The filter setting was set at 1-30 Hz and at least 150 sweeps were obtained for each trial.

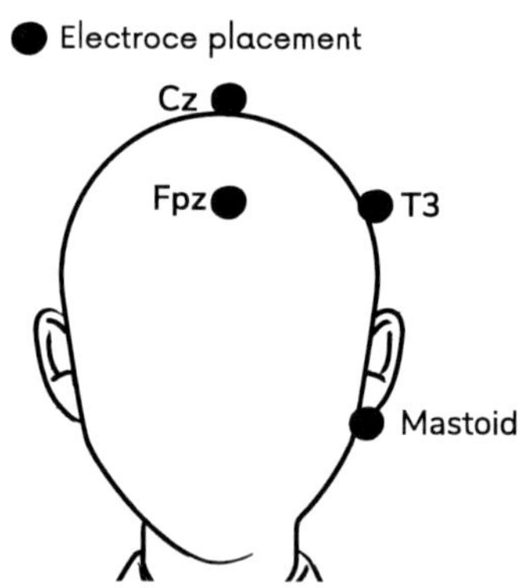

Figure 1. The placement of electrodes in cortical auditory evoked potential (CAEP) recording (C_Z versus T_3)

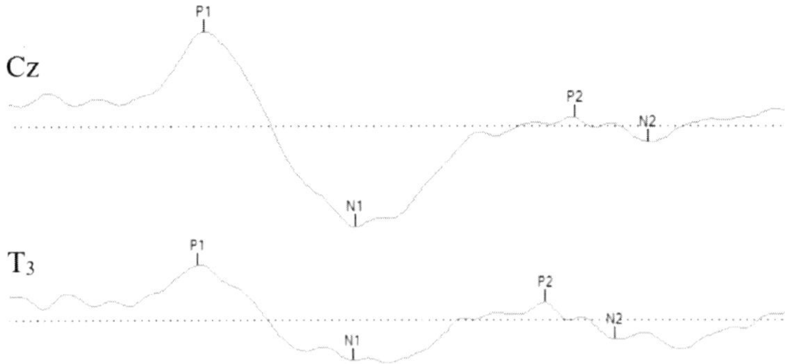

Figure 2. The prominent peaks of cortical auditory evoked potential (CAEP) waveforms (elicited by /ba/ stimulus) recorded at Cz and T_3 electrode placements.

Table 1. Comparisons of cortical auditory evoked potential (CAEP) results between Cz and T_3 electrode placements

Latency (ms)	CZ				T3			
	P1	N1	P2	N2	P1	N1	P2	N2
/ba/	149.9	262.3	424.7		146.0	245.7	362.3	372.7
/m/	135.3	237.4	391.4	453.9	127.0	218.6	358.1	410.2
/g/	139.5	235.3	356.0	393.5	129.1	231.1	360.2	399.8
/t/	135.3	231.1	368.5	418.5	131.2	235.3	366.4	458.1
Amplitude (μV)	CZ				T3			
	P1	N1	P2	N2	P1	N1	P2	N2
/ba/	5.9	8.4	2.6		2.6	4.1	1.2	0.2
/m/	7.7	7.3	2.4	0.6	5.2	2.2	0.3	2.9
/g/	5.5	8.6	3.0	0.8	3.4	4.9	2.4	1.6
/t/	9.7	10.3	0.9	1.7	5.9	4.2	1.9	3.0

The resultant CAEP peaks were identified and plotted (within a time window of -50 to 700 ms) by two experts in the field of electrophysiology by agreement. Figure 2 depicts the aided CAEP waveforms (evoked by /ba/ stimulus), with Table 1 displaying absolute latency and amplitude values of P_1, N_1, P_2, and N_2 peaks (elicited by 4 speech stimuli) for each electrode montage. In general, the morphology of waveforms was good and the prominent peaks (P_1, N_1, P_2 and, N_2) were identifiable for each stimulus. As shown in Table 1, relative to the T_3 electrode montage, the amplitudes of most CAEP peaks were descriptively higher for the Cz location. On the other hand, the T_3 electrode location produced CAEP peaks with mostly shorter latencies than the Cz electrode montage.

Discussion

In normal hearing listeners, the auditory cortex matures in response to age and auditory inputs. It may differ from hearing-impaired children who might receive inadequate auditory responses since birth. In this case report, clear and repeatable CAEP waveforms were obtained for each stimulus. This finding is expected as the speech stimuli were presented at a comfortable intensity level (65 dB SPL) and the hearing aids were functioning well during the CAEP testing. The consistent use of hearing aids may also contribute to reasonably robust CAEP responses (13).

When the two electrode montages were compared, it was found that the aided CAEP responses exhibited greater amplitudes for the Cz location (in comparison to the T_3 location) for all speech stimuli. On the other hand, as reported by Wunderlich et al. (14), the T_3 electrode montage was preferred because of its larger CAEP waveforms than the Cz location. The disagreement between the studies is that in this case report, the hearing of the child was abnormal (despite the fact that the free-field aided responses were within the speech spectrum), while Wunderlich et al. (14) measured CAEP responses from normal-hearing children. There are limitations when comparing the CAEP waveforms of hearing-impaired children with their normal peers (from anatomical and pathophysiological perspectives). The Cz electrode montage has been suggested to be the preferred electrode montage in developing the basic foundation for clinical applications. However, only a limited set of normative values based on various stimuli are currently available and are not used in the CAEP testing in clinical settings.

In terms of audibility and behavioral benefit from amplification, this child demonstrated age-appropriate outcomes that should aid in the central maturation. However, weaker left temporal responses are likely to reflect ongoing functional delays in cortical areas associated with linguistic processing (16), whereas robust midline activity indicates accurate signal detection. These performance-neurophysiological dissociations have been well documented in hearing aid and cochlear implant users with residual language impairments, despite interventions that improve sound access (17). This case report reinforces the notion that localized, electrode dependent CAEP characteristics may provide additional information about the central auditory status beyond audibility measures alone.

Specifically, the T_3 electrode location reveals functional specialization of posterior superior temporal areas important for speech-language advancement (18). The midline Cz electrode, on the other hand, focuses on cortical processes that are required in primary auditory regions only. Thus, relying solely on the Cz position risks overlooking higher-order maturation, which is critical for real-world listening. While the Cz location confirms audibility as a starting point for improvement, incorporating temporal channels (T_3 location) assesses the efficacy of amplifying access to speech elements and corresponding cognitive skills over time.

Collectively, this case report emphasizes the importance of multi-electrode recording in accurately determining the central benefit of intervention by exposing differential neural activity related to both low-level signal detection and higher linguistic functions. Tailoring CAEP electrode montages to distinguish sensory and cognitive subprocesses increases dimensionality for tracing pediatric auditory development with the use of hearing amplification devices.

Conclusion

The multi-electrode recording of CAEP is beneficial to distinguish basic sensory improvements from higher-order cognitive gains in an aided hearing-impaired child. While the Cz location confirms the presence of amplified signals, the temporal location indicates the maturation of speech-language networks. The findings in this case report indicate that the standard CAEP protocols should include both midline and lateral electrodes. Differentiating signal access from functional development allows for targeted rehabilitation of residual deficits in hearing device users. The use of electrode montages that expose distinct neural processes would allow for more precise assessments of intervention benefits to promote auditory development in children.

Declaration of patient consent

The authors certify that they have obtained the consent form from the patient. In the form, the patient has given her consent for her image and other clinical information to be reported in the journal. The patient understands that her name and initial will not be published, and due efforts will be made to conceal her identity, but anonymity cannot be guaranteed.

References

[1] Romli M, Wan Mohamad WN, Awang MA, Aw CL, Zakaria MN. The clinical value of bilateral bone conduction testing in hearing diagnosis. Indian J Otol 2020;26(3):182-5.

[2] Abdul Wahab NA, Wahab S, Abdul Rahman AH, Sidek D, Zakaria MN. The hyperactivity of efferent auditory system in patients with schizophrenia: a transient evoked otoacoustic emissions study. Psychiatr Investig 2016;13(1):82-8.

[3] Wahab S, Zakaria MN, Sidek D, Abdul Rahman AH, Shah SA, Abdul Wahab NA. Evaluation of auditory hallucinations in patients with schizophrenia: A validation study of the Malay version of Psychotic Symptom Rating Scales (PSYRATS). Psychiatr Res 2015;228(3):462-7.

[4] Wong JW, Wan Mohamad WN, Wan Husain WS, Zakaria MN. The tinnitus suppressive effect: Comparisons between three types of maskers. Int J Disabil Hum Dev 2020;19(1):21-6.

[5] Zakaria MN. The effectiveness of sound therapy in treating patients with mild and severe tinnitus. Int J Disabil Hum Dev 2020;19(2):215-9.

[6] Wan Mohamad WN, Romli M, Awang MA, Abdullah R, Lih AC, Zakaria MN. The presence of unusual bone conduction thresholds in pure tone audiometry. Indian J Otol 2020;26(1):54-7.

[7] Lih AC, Zakaria MN, Mohamad RA, Nor Rashid MF. Effects of ethnicity and gender on the middle ear function in Asian adults. Indian J Otol 2017;23(2):94-7.

[8] Katz J, Marshall C, English K, Hood L, Tillery KL. Handbook of clinical audiology. Philadelphia: Lippincott Williams Wilkins, 2015.

[9] Hall JW. New handbook of auditory evoked responses. Boston, MA: Pearson, 2007.

[10] Mukari SZS, Umat C, Chan SC, Ali A, Maamor N, Zakaria MN. Effects of age and type of stimulus on the cortical auditory evoked potential in healthy Malaysian children. J Audiol Otol 2020;24(1):35-9.

[11] Sharma A, Martin K, Roland P, Bauer P, Sweeney MH, Gilley P, et al. P1 latency as a biomarker for central auditory development in children with hearing impairment. J Am Acad Audiol 2005;16(8):564-73.

[12] Billings CJ, Papesh MA, Penman TM, Baltzell LS, Gallun FJ. Clinical use of aided cortical auditory evoked potentials as a measure of physiological detection or physiological discrimination. Int J Otolaryngol 2012;2012:365752.

[13] Ching TY, Zhang VW, Hou S, Van Buynder P. Cortical auditory evoked potentials reveal changes in audibility with nonlinear frequency compression in hearing aids for children: clinical implications. Semin Hear 2016;37(1):25-35.

[14] Wunderlich JL, Cone-Wesson BK, Shepherd R. Maturation of the cortical auditory evoked potential in infants and young children. Hear Res 2006;212(1-2):185-202.

[15] Tomé D, Barbosa F, Nowak K, Marques-Teixeira J. The development of the N1 and N2 components in auditory oddball paradigms: a systematic review with narrative analysis and suggested normative values. J Neural Transm (Vienna) 2015;122(3):375-91.

[16] Chang HW, Dillon H, Carter L, van Dun B, Young ST. The relationship between cortical auditory evoked potential (CAEP) detection and estimated audibility in infants with sensorineural hearing loss. Int J Audiol 2012;51(9):663-70.

[17] McCreery RW, Walker EA, Spratford M, Bentler R, Holte L, Roush P, et al. Longitudinal Predictors of Aided Speech Audibility in Infants and Children. Ear Hear 2015;36 Suppl 1(0 1):24S-37S.

[18] Alvarenga KF, Amorim RB, Agostinho-Pesse RS, Costa OA, Nascimento LT, Bevilacqua MC. Speech perception and cortical auditory evoked potentials in cochlear implant users with auditory neuropathy spectrum disorders. Int J Pediatr Otorhinolaryngol 2012;76(9):1332-8.

Chapter 17

Pure tone audiometry (PTA) and diagnosing hearing problems

Mohd N Zakaria, PhD
Audiology Programme, School of Health Sciences, Universiti Sains Malaysia, Kelantan, Malaysia

Abstract

Pure tone audiometry (PTA) has been regarded as the gold standard test for diagnosing hearing problems. In this test, air conduction (AC) and bone conduction (BC) thresholds are determined so that the severity of hearing loss, as well as the type of hearing loss, can be documented. Due to reported problems (such as acoustic radiation), the BC testing is usually limited to frequencies not more than 4000 Hz. In this chapter, we highlight the need to have a BC threshold at 6000 Hz (to make an accurate hearing diagnosis), and this threshold can be reliable enough to be taken into consideration (despite having some issues). Depending on the case, it appears worthwhile to measure the 6000 Hz BC threshold, and if this turns out to be problematic, certain measures can be taken to support the PTA results.

Introduction

Humans are blessed with optimal hearing function, which is crucial for effective engagement in daily interactions and tasks (1). This being said, impairment of the auditory system may result in hearing deficiency and associated manifestations (2-6). Numerous adverse consequences can result from untreated hearing loss when not accurately diagnosed and treated. The

In: Public Health: Audiology Research in Malaysia
Editors: Mohd N. Zakaria and Joav Merrick
ISBN: 979-8-89530-577-5

extent of hearing difficulties experienced is contingent upon the severity of the hearing impairment, which can vary from mild to profound (1). Meanwhile, the three primary categories of hearing impairment include conductive hearing loss (CHL), sensorineural hearing loss (SNHL), and mixed hearing loss (MHL) (1). In view of this, it is essential to acquire precise assessments of hearing in order to facilitate prompt implementation of suitable treatment and/or intervention.

The assessment of hearing function is commonly conducted through the use of pure tone audiometry (PTA) (2). This diagnostic clinical procedure involves the determination of air conduction (AC) and bone conduction (BC) thresholds at specified frequencies. The results of these thresholds, as depicted on an audiogram, serve to indicate the degree of hearing impairment and the type of the hearing loss (2). For instance, in cases of CHL, individuals exhibit normal BC thresholds (≤ 20 dB HL) but abnormal AC thresholds (exceeding 20 dB HL), along with significant air-bone gaps (ABGs). Conversely, SNHL is characterized by abnormal AC and BC thresholds without the presence of ABGs. Moreover, in cases of MHL, significant ABGs are observed, and both AC and BC thresholds fall outside the normal range (1).

While the AC thresholds can be conveniently determined at various frequencies (i.e., up to 8000 Hz with the conventional audiometer), the BC thresholds are typically measured at frequencies not more than 4000 Hz. Comparatively, the BC testing is known to have more "problems" (relative to the AC testing), which is primarily related to the design of the bone vibrator used (7-12). In this regard, confirming the type of hearing loss can be problematic if the BC thresholds are not available at certain frequencies. As such, this paper highlights the usefulness of having the BC threshold at 6000 Hz (despite it not being the recommended standard) in order to achieve an accurate hearing diagnosis.

Case report

Audiological evaluations were conducted on a 41-year-old Malay man with a main complaint of continuous high-pitched tinnitus in his left ear. The tinnitus started approximately 6 months ago, and he found it to be disturbing and annoying. He also could not sleep well due to the constant ringing sound. The possible cause of his tinnitus was unknown. He indicated having good hearing in both ears and did not experience difficulties listening to conversations (either in quiet or noisy environments). Previously employed as a healthcare assistant for a period of three years, his duties involved frequent exposure to a loud fogging machine for mosquito control. There were no reports of otalgia, otorrhea, or otological diseases. Additionally, he was in overall good health with no other medical conditions noted.

The otoscopic examination found him to have an intact tympanic membrane and a clear ear canal for each ear. According to the recommended testing procedures (13-15), he underwent several other assessments, including tympanometry, acoustic reflex, and PTA. His middle ear status was assessed using a 226 Hz tympanometer (GSI TympStar Pro, Grason-Stadler Inc., USA), revealing normal function indicated by a type A tympanogram for each ear. Additionally, normal ipsilateral acoustic reflex thresholds (ranging from 70-100 dB) were observed at 500 Hz, 1000 Hz, and 2000 Hz frequencies. Subsequently, his hearing was evaluated using a two-channel audiometer (GSI 61, Grason-Stadler Inc., USA), The TDH-39 headphone and B71 bone vibrator were used to document AC and BC thresholds, respectively. For each ear, the AC thresholds are measured at 250, 500, 1000, 2000, 3000, 4000, 6000, and 8000 Hz, while the BC thresholds are assessed at 250, 500, 1000, 2000, and 4000 Hz. His PTA results are depicted in Figure 1. As shown, he was found to have normal hearing in the right ear, with the exception of a mild loss at 8000 Hz. On the other hand, his left ear showed mild to moderate hearing loss (starting from 2000 Hz and onwards, with other frequencies being within the normal range). In addition, a notch at 6000 Hz for the BC threshold was noted.

By considering the available PTA findings, it is noteworthy to highlight that the type of hearing loss could not be confirmed, particularly for the left ear. The left BC thresholds were all within the normal limits (i.e., from 250 to 4000 Hz). In fact, a more prominent hearing loss was actually observed at 6000 Hz, but the diagnosis could not be completed as there was no BC threshold. Even though tympanometry and acoustic reflex results may suggest the absence of CHL, getting evidence from the audiogram is still necessary. In view of this, it was then decided to proceed with the BC testing at this particular frequency. As revealed in Figure 1, the unmasked BC thresholds at 6000 Hz were 15 dB HL and 10 dB HL for the left and right ears, respectively. An appropriate masking procedure was then performed to obtain the masked BC threshold for the left ear. This procedure was indeed successful, and the left masked BC threshold at 6000 Hz was plotted at 45 dB HL. Based on this additional result, the type of hearing loss for the left ear could now be confirmed (i.e., SNHL).

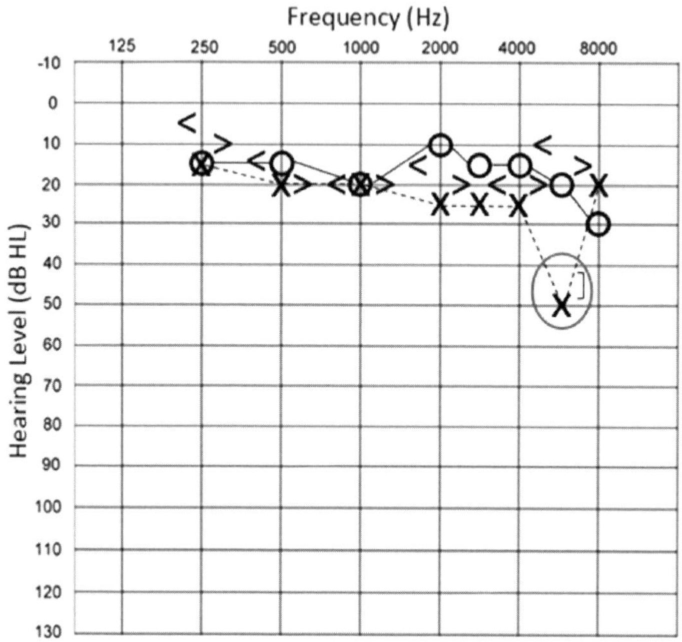

Figure 1. Pure tone audiometry (PTA) results of the patient.

Discussion

Even though the PTA testing has been commonly used for diagnosing the degree and type of hearing loss, it does have some issues worthy of being highlighted (7-12). Information from BC thresholds (in addition to AC thresholds) is imperative in order to make a decision on the type of hearing loss (7-12). Ensuring a precise diagnosis of hearing impairment is crucial for the effective implementation of tailored treatment strategies (1).

In the BC testing, the frequencies to be tested are more limited (relative to the AC testing), i.e., from 250 to 4000 Hz. There are several reasons why assessing BC thresholds at higher frequencies (beyond 4000 Hz) can be problematic (1, 10, 11). One frequently debated issue is the potential impact of acoustic radiation. By definition, acoustic radiation refers to the emission of sound energy from a bone vibrator utilized in bone conduction testing, which can be picked up by the air conduction system. The existence of acoustic radiation can lead to false BC thresholds (better than they should be), contributing to questionable ABGs, particularly at high frequencies (10, 11).

In a study by Lightfoot and Hughes (10) involving 20 normal-hearing adults, ABGs at 3000 Hz, 4000 Hz, 6000 Hz, and 8000 Hz were investigated. As reported, in the unoccluded ear condition, the mean ABGs could be as high as 18.8 dB. For example, at 4000 Hz and 6000 Hz frequencies, the mean ABGs were 5.3 dB and 18.8 dB, respectively. When the ear was occluded (e.g., by using earphones), reduced mean ABGs were observed (i.e., 4.5 dB and 14.8 dB at 4000 Hz and 6000 Hz, respectively). Herein, by occluding the ear, the impact of the acoustic radiation was minimized. Other possible factors that contributed to the large ABGs were calibration errors and the design of bone vibrators (10). Due to this, the BC testing at frequencies greater than 4000 Hz should be avoided, and this recommendation has been universally accepted in clinical practice. In line with this, some studies found that the false ABGs could also occur at 4000 Hz, which was likely due to calibration issues (rather than acoustic radiation (11, 12).

In this case report, it is noted that the inclusion of the 6000 Hz BC threshold, while not typically recommended, can be beneficial for confirming the type of hearing loss in the patient's left ear (i.e., SNHL). Considering the aforementioned issue, the worse-case scenario is that a large ABG should have been noted at this frequency (resulting in a diagnosis of either CHL or MHL). However, a reliable BC threshold was in fact obtained. In view of this, assessing the BC threshold at 6000 Hz is still a viable option (perhaps it is not a good idea to fully disregard this). This being said, if it turns out to be problematic, the hearing diagnosis can still be established by integrating all audiological findings. For his right ear, the majority of the frequencies revealed normal AC and BC thresholds. Even though there was a mild hearing loss at 8000 Hz, the type of hearing loss was likely to be SNHL (and the BC testing was not carried out at this frequency due to notable calibration errors and the impact of acoustic radiation). In terms of case management, the patient was referred to a specialized tinnitus clinic to manage his disturbing tinnitus.

Conclusion

Clinically, getting an accurate hearing diagnosis (including the degree of hearing loss and the type of hearing loss) for every patient is crucial. As shown in this paper, even though it is not a common practice, measuring the BC threshold beyond 4000 Hz (i.e., at least at 6000 Hz) can be useful and imperative for confirming the type of hearing loss. Should any issue arise, certain measures can be taken to support the PTA results.

Declaration of patient consent

The authors certify that they have obtained the consent form from the patient. In the form, the patient has given his consent for his image and other clinical information to be reported in the journal. The patient understands that his name and initial will not be published, and due efforts will be made to conceal his identity, but anonymity cannot be guaranteed.

References

[1] Katz J, Marshall C, English K, Hood L, Tillery KL. Handbook of clinical audiology. Philadelphia: Lippincott Williams Wilkins, 2015.

[2] Wan Mohamad WN, Romli M, Awang MA, Abdullah R, Lih AC, Zakaria MN. The presence of unusual bone conduction thresholds in pure tone audiometry. Indian J Otol 2020;26(1):54-7.

[3] Zainun Z, Zakaria MN, Sidek D, Ismail Z. Clinical use of Malay version of vertigo symptom scale (MWSS) in patients with peripheral vestibular disorder (PVD). Med J Malaysia 2012;67(4):386-9.

[4] Wong JW, Wan Mohamad WN, Wan Husain WS, Zakaria MN. The tinnitus suppressive effect: Comparisons between three types of maskers. Int J Disabil Hum Dev 2020;19(1):21-6.

[5] Zakaria MN. The effectiveness of sound therapy in treating patients with mild and severe tinnitus. Int J Disabil Hum Dev 2020;19(2):215-9.

[6] Abdul Wahab NA, Wahab S, Abdul Rahman AH, Sidek D, Zakaria MN. The hyperactivity of efferent auditory system in patients with schizophrenia: a transient evoked otoacoustic emissions study. Psychiatry Investig 2016;13(1):82-8.

[7] Eichenauer A, Dillon H, Clinch B, Loi T. Effect of bone-conduction harmonic distortions on hearing thresholds. J Acoust Soc Am 2014;136(2):EL96-102.

[8] Fröhlich L, Plontke SK, Rahne T. Influence of transducer types on bone conduction hearing thresholds. PLoS One 2018;13:e0195233.

[9] Jansson KJ, Håkansson B, Johannsen L, Tengstrand T. Electro-acoustic performance of the new bone vibrator radioear B81: A comparison with the conventional radioear B71. Int J Audiol 2015;54:334-40.

[10] Lightfoot GR, Hughes JB. Bone conduction errors at high frequencies: Implications for clinical and medico-legal practice J Laryngol Otol 1993;107: 305-8.

[11] Tate Maltby M, Gaszczyk D. Is it necessary to occlude the ear in bone-conduction testing at 4 kHz, in order to prevent air-borne radiation affecting the results? Int J Audiol 2015;54:918-23.

[12] Margolis RH, Eikelboom RH, Johnson C, Ginter SM, Swanepoel de W, Moore BC. False air-bone gaps at 4 kHz in listeners with normal hearing and sensorineural hearing loss. Int J Audiol 2013;52(8):526-32.

[13] Romli M, Wan Mohamad WN, Awang MA, Aw CL, Zakaria MN. The clinical value of bilateral bone conduction testing in hearing diagnosis. Indian J Otol 2020;26(3):182-5.
[14] Lih AC, Zakaria MN, Mohamad RA, Nor Rashid MF. Effects of ethnicity and gender on the middle ear function in Asian adults. Indian J Otol 2017;23(2):94-7.
[15] Awang MA, Zakaria MN. Acoustic reflex testing in clinical audiology: What is the next direction? Int J Disabil Hum Dev 2019;18(2):123-8.

Chapter 18

Understanding the relationship between cochlear implant (CI) mapping and cortical auditory evoked potential (CAEP)

Rosninda Abdullah[1], MSc
Noor AA Wahab[1], PhD
Nashrah Maamor[2], PhD
Nik AN Othman[3], MMed
Basyariatul F Othman[2], PhD
and Mohd N Zakaria[4], PhD

[1]Audiology Programme, Centre for Rehabilitation and Special Needs Studies, Faculty of Health Sciences, Universiti Kebangsaan Malaysia, Kuala Lumpur, Malaysia
[2]Centre for Ear, Hearing and Speech, Faculty of Health Sciences, Universiti Kebangsaan Malaysia, Kuala Lumpur, Malaysia
[3]Department of Otorhinolaryngology, School of Medical Sciences, Universiti Sains Malaysia, Kelantan, Malaysia, and [4]Audiology Programme, School of Health Sciences, Universiti Sains Malaysia, Kelantan, Malaysia

Abstract

The cortical auditory evoked potential (CAEP) is an objective test that can be used to measure the benefit of cochlear implants (CIs) in adults and children. In this chapter, we present a complex case of a 12-year-old Malay girl CI recipient who was born with Pendred syndrome and had progressive asymmetrical sensorineural hearing loss. We aim to share our experience in verifying the most comfortable level (MCL) of the CI device using the CAEP assessment, which was conducted in two sessions, i.e., before and after remapping. In this case, the child was

In: Public Health: Audiology Research in Malaysia
Editors: Mohd N. Zakaria and Joav Merrick
ISBN: 979-8-89530-577-5

unable to accurately judge the loudness of the stimulated channels during the conventional behavioural mapping, which also showed poor CAEP responses. Subsequently, the CI device was remapped using the electrically evoked stapedial reflex threshold (ESRT) approach. In addition to improved aided free-field thresholds, more robust CAEP waveforms were observed after the remapping procedure. Most of the CAEP peaks showed larger amplitudes and shorter latencies as a result of the ESRT-based map. This case report demonstrates the feasibility and usefulness of CAEP in verifying the CI mapping in a complex case.

Introduction

The preservation of optimal auditory function is crucial for the execution of everyday activities. The onset of auditory impairments, including hearing loss, can substantially compromise the quality of life of those affected (1). As such, it is of utmost importance to conduct comprehensive auditory evaluations to accurately diagnose hearing impairments (2-5). Based on the hearing diagnosis (i.e., type of loss and severity of hearing loss), tailored treatment and intervention approaches are provided to those suffering from hearing loss (1).

For children and adults who are diagnosed with severe or profound hearing loss (due to damage to the inner ear), cochlear implants (CIs) are recommended (6, 7). This device consists of two main parts. The first part is an external unit, positioned behind the ear, which houses a microphone. This microphone captures acoustic signals and transforms them into electrical signals. These electrical signals are then relayed to the second component of the device, an internal part that is surgically implanted beneath the skin, usually behind the ear or in the neck. The internal part of CI is connected to an electrode array. This electrode array transmits the respective electrical impulses directly to the auditory nerve, thereby stimulating the higher levels of the auditory system, up to and including the auditory cortex (for sound interpretation) (1). As demonstrated elsewhere, CIs have been found to be effective in improving auditory, speech, and language skills in paediatric CI recipients (8-10).

When the CI device is fitted and switched on, a mapping procedure must be conducted (1, 6). In this regard, it is crucial to establish the electrical dynamic range (EDR) of each CI electrode by determining the minimum (T level) and maximum comfortable level (MCL) when stimulating the auditory nerve without causing discomfort. The CI programming procedure is typically conducted using subjective psychoacoustic responses, which may increase the risk of under- or over-stimulation, especially in complex cases (6). To address this, objective measures can be considered in the CI mapping (1, 6, 11-14). In line with this, a non-invasive cortical auditory evoked potential (CAEP) is an emerging technique that can be employed to objectively verify CI mapping in adults (15, 16) and children (17,18). In this paper, we aim to share our experience in verifying the MCL of a complex paediatric case using the CAEP testing (conducted before and after remapping of the CI device).

Case report

A 12-year-old Malay girl with Pendred syndrome, central hypothyroidism, and progressive asymmetrical SNHL came to the Audiology Clinic, University Hospital, for audiological evaluations. She was diagnosed to have profound SNHL in the right ear and moderate to severe SNHL in the left ear when she was 3 years of age. Following this, she was fitted with behind-the-ear (BTE) hearing aids (Bernafon Supremia 3) bilaterally. Due to the nature of her hearing loss (i.e., progressive), she can communicate using spoken language and attends a mainstream school.

Approximately two years after using the binaural hearing aids, she received a CI device (Nucleus Profile CI522) for her right ear. The switch on of her CI was conducted based on the post-operative electrically evoked compound action potential (ECAP) thresholds. However, she reported difficulties to appreciate sounds produced by the CI device. Due to this, attempts were made to remap the CI according to her subjective psychoacoustic responses in the subsequent follow-ups. Because she was unable to give proper loudness and pitch judgment, the electrically evoked stapedial reflex threshold (ESRT) approach was then conducted to remap her CI device objectively (by changing MCL settings).

Figure 1 shows the patient's aided free-field thresholds before and after the remapping procedure (with the ESRT method). In this free-field test, a calibrated two-channel audiometer (GSI 61, Grason-Stadler Inc., USA) was used, and pure tones were delivered via a loudspeaker. As illustrated, after remapping her CI device, the aided thresholds improved notably across the speech spectrum (approaching normal-hearing limits). This demonstrates the usefulness of having the ESRT-based map when the behavioural map is questionable or not optimized.

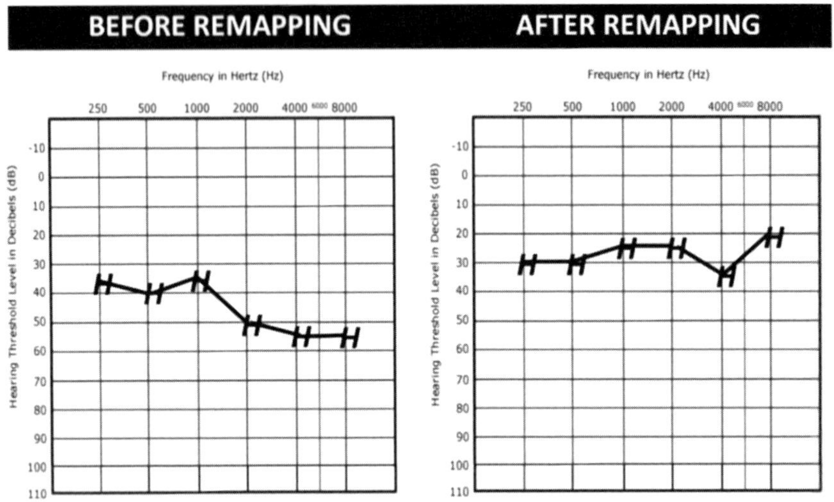

Figure 1. Comparisons of aided free-field test results of the patient before and after the remapping procedure (with the electrically evoked stapedial reflex threshold method).

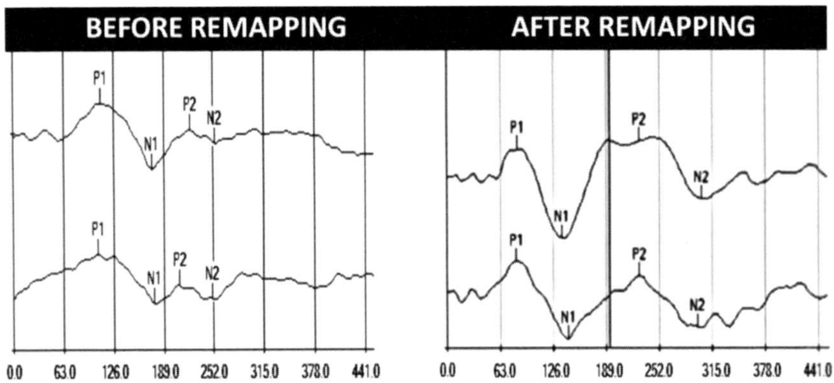

Figure 2. Comparisons of cortical auditory evoked potential (CAEP) waveforms of the patient before and after the remapping procedure (with the electrically evoked stapedial reflex threshold method).

The patient also underwent the CAEP testing twice, i.e., before and after the remapping of the CI device (with the ESRT technique). The testing was carried out in a soundproof room, and the Biologic Navigator Pro AEP device was employed to record the required waveforms. To capture CAEP responses, the inverting electrode was placed at the Cz location, the non-inverting electrode at the mastoid (M1), and the common electrode at the high forehead

(Fpz) location. The impedance of the electrodes was maintained below 5 kΩ during the measurement.

The stimulus for eliciting CAEP waveforms was the speech syllable /ba/ (70 ms in duration). The stimulus was presented repetitively at a stimulus rate of 1.1/s through a loudspeaker placed at 0° azimuth while the child sat comfortably and watched a silent movie (with minimal eye blinking). The intensity level was set at 65 dB SPL. The resulting waveforms were bandpass filtered between 1 and 30 Hz, and 200 sweeps were obtained for each trial.

Figure 2 illustrates the child's CAEP results recorded in the two sessions. As revealed, more robust CAEP waveforms were observed after the remapping process. Herein, most of the CAEP peaks showed larger amplitudes and shorter latencies as a result of the ESRT-based map. In the first session, P1, N1, and P2 peaks were elicited at 95.8 ms, 168.6 ms, and 268.6 ms, respectively. After the remapping procedure, the latencies became shorter (i.e., 78.1 ms, 166.6 ms, and 220.7 ms for P1, N1, and P2, respectively). Likewise, the amplitudes increased from 0.1 μV to 3.4 μV for P1, 1.6 μV to 3.5 μV for N1, and from 1.5 μV to 2.3 μV for P2. These findings clearly demonstrate how appropriate map settings of the CI device can improve hearing and speech perception.

Of note, the child also reported better audibility with the new map, which is consistent with improved aided free-field aided thresholds and CAEP findings. She was advised to continue using both the CI and the hearing aid to maximize her auditory exposure and experience. Her hearing status will also be monitored from time to time (and further remapping is necessary if her hearing levels change over time).

Discussion

Nowadays, there are various treatment options for hearing loss cases (1). With the emergence of CI, children and adults with profound hearing loss can be managed and intervened appropriately. Providing sufficient amplification to hearing-impaired children is undoubtedly important to foster adequate speech and language development. Following the CI surgery, the CI device must be programmed (by determining the T level and MCL for each CI electrode). This mapping procedure is typically conducted using subjective measures, which can be affected by several factors, including patients' condition and cooperation (1, 6).

The child in this case report was diagnosed with Pendred syndrome (with hypothyroidism) and progressive hearing loss. As reported elsewhere, the progressive hearing loss is indeed one of the common features of those with Pendred syndrome (19, 20). Similar to this case report, the hearing levels of children with this syndrome could worsen and reach profound deafness (21). Studies have also demonstrated the benefits of having CIs for severe to profound hearing-impaired children with Pendred syndrome (22, 23).

Given that the hearing loss is progressive in nature, she is able to speak properly, and has been attending the mainstream school. This is rather sensible, as she might have had normal hearing (or mild hearing loss) before and acquired sufficient speech and language skills. Nevertheless, she had difficulties reporting the optimum MCL for the tested CI electrodes after many attempts (and this could be due to her medical conditions). In line with this, children with hypothyroidism have been reported to be at risk of having auditory processing deficits and cognitive problems (24, 25).

Because the behavioural mapping approach was unsuccessful, an alternative approach should be considered. Her CI device was then remapped using the ESRT method. This mapping technique was chosen for several reasons. First, it is an objective measure, which is suitable in cases where the behavioural mapping method is challenging or produces questionable results (1, 6). Second, it can be administered conveniently using the existing immittance audiometric device with a simple protocol (6). Lastly, it has been proven to be useful in predicting MCLs in children with CIs (leading to improved CI outcomes) (12, 26, 27).

As clearly shown, positive outcomes were noted after applying the ESRT-based map for this patient. In particular, notable improvements were seen in the free-field aided test. Herein, it is rather expected to see better hearing thresholds when the MCL was increased (to the level that did cause over-amplification or discomfort). The decision to change the map settings could not be made before, as the child was unable to give reliable reports. Likewise, more robust CAEP waveforms were observed following the remapping process. Having CAEP responses with larger amplitudes and shorter latencies indicates enhanced neural firing, and that the auditory information has been optimally perceived by the auditory cortex for further processing (1, 11). This finding is in line with a study by Kosaner et al. (18) that used the ESRT-based map and found good CAEP responses in CI users.

Conclusion

This chapter highlights the benefit of having the CAEP testing in verifying the CI mapping in a difficult case (objectively). Additionally, the ESRT approach is useful in providing sufficient MCLs (where the behavioural map is questionable) to enhance auditory exposure and experience. With a simple equipment setup, the CAEP testing can be conveniently conducted in clinical practice. The results gathered could assist clinicians in better understanding how the brain responds to various CI map settings and could be useful during counselling sessions.

Declaration of patient consent

The authors certify that they have obtained the consent form from the patient or her guardian. In the form, the patient or her guardian has given consent for her image and other clinical information to be reported in the journal. The patient or her guardian understands that her name and initial will not be published, and due efforts will be made to conceal her identity, but anonymity cannot be guaranteed.

References

[1] Katz J, Marshall C, English K, Hood L, Tillery KL. Handbook of clinical audiology. Philadelphia: Lippincott Williams Wilkins, 2015.

[2] Romli M, Wan Mohamad WN, Awang MA, Aw CL, Zakaria MN. The clinical value of bilateral bone conduction testing in hearing diagnosis. Indian J Otol 2020;26(3):182-5.

[3] Lih AC, Zakaria MN, Mohamad RA, Nor Rashid MF. Effects of ethnicity and gender on the middle ear function in Asian adults. Indian J Otol 2017;23(2):94-7.

[4] Abdul Wahab NA, Wahab S, Abdul Rahman AH, Sidek D, Zakaria MN. The hyperactivity of efferent auditory system in patients with schizophrenia: a transient evoked otoacoustic emissions study. Psychiatry Investig 2016;13(1):82-8.

[5] Jalaei B, Azmi MHAM, Zakaria MN. Gender differences in binaural speech-evoked auditory brainstem response: are they clinically significant? Braz J Otorhinolaryngol 2019;85(4):486-93.

[6] Aw CL, Tan SK, Abdullah R, Othman NAN, Zakaria MN. Electrically evoked stapedial reflex threshold assessment among Malaysian cochlear implant users: Comparisons between different stimulus rates. Indian J Otol 2020;26(2):89-92.

[7] Hassan MNHC, Mohamad WNW, Awang MA, Maamor N, Wahab NAA, Zakaria MN. Does the auditory localization ability improve with the use of cochlear implant? Int J Disabil Hum Dev 2021;20(3):237-42.

[8] Bond M, Mealing S, Anderson R, Elston J, Weiner G, Taylor RS, et al. The effectiveness and cost-effectiveness of cochlear implants for severe to profound deafness in children and adults: a systematic review and economic model. Health Technol Assess 2009;13(44):1-330.

[9] Sharma SD, Cushing SL, Papsin BC, Gordon KA. Hearing and speech benefits of cochlear implantation in children: A review of the literature. Int J Pediatr Otorhinolaryngol 2020;133:109984.

[10] Langman AW, Quigley SM, Souliere CR Jr. Cochlear implants in children. Pediatr Clin North Am 1996;43:1217-31.

[11] Hall JW. New handbook of auditory evoked responses. Boston, MA: Pearson, 2007.

[12] Kosaner J, Spitzer P, Bayguzina S, Gultekin M, Behar LA. Comparing eSRT and eCAP measurements in pediatric MED-EL cochlear implant users. Cochlear Implants Int 2018;19(3):153-161.

[13] Wang Y, Pan T, Deshpande SB, Ma F. The relationship between eABR and auditory performance and speech intelligibility outcomes in pediatric cochlear implant recipients. Am J Audiol 2015;24(2):226-34.

[14] Mukari SZS, Umat C, Chan SC, Ali A, Maamor N, Zakaria MN. Effects of age and type of stimulus on the cortical auditory evoked potential in healthy Malaysian children. J Audiol Otol 2020;24(1):35-9.

[15] Liebscher T, Alberter K, Hoppe U. Cortical auditory evoked potentials in cochlear implant listeners via single electrode stimulation in relation to speech perception. Int J Audiol 2018;57(12):933-40.

[16] Távora-Vieira D, Mandruzzato G, Polak M, Truong B, Stutley A. Comparative analysis of cortical auditory evoked potential in cochlear implant users. Ear Hear 2021;42(6):1755-69.

[17] Silva LA, Couto MI, Tsuji RK, Bento RF, de Carvalho AC, Matas CG. Auditory cortical maturation in a child with cochlear implant: analysis of electrophysiological and behavioral measures. Case Rep Otolaryngol 2015;2015:890508.

[18] Kosaner J, Van Dun B, Yigit O, Gultekin M, Bayguzina S. Clinically recorded cortical auditory evoked potentials from paediatric cochlear implant users fitted with electrically elicited stapedius reflex thresholds. Int J Pediatr Otorhinolaryngol 2018;108:100-12.

[19] Cremers CW, Admiraal RJ, Huygen PL, Bolder C, Everett LA, Joosten FB, et al. Progressive hearing loss, hypoplasia of the cochlea and widened vestibular aqueducts are very common features in Pendred's syndrome. Int J Pediatr Otorhinolaryngol 1998;45(2):113-23.

[20] Mey K, Bille M, Rye Rasmussen SH, Tranebjærg L, Cayé-Thomasen P. The natural history of hearing loss in Pendred syndrome and non-syndromic enlarged vestibular aqueduct. Otol Neurotol 2019;40(3):e178-e185.

[21] Lado Abeal J. Pendred syndrome. Expert Rev Endocrinol Metab 2008;3(5):635-43.

[22] van Nierop JW, Huinck WJ, Pennings RJ, Admiraal RJ, Mylanus EA, Kunst HP. Patients with Pendred syndrome: is cochlear implantation beneficial? Clin Otolaryngol 2016;41(4):386-94.

[23] Patterson TE, Gonzalez VB, Carron JD. Cochlear implantation in patients with Pendred syndrome. Am J Otolaryngol 2021;42(6):103087.

[24] Diaz A, Lipman Diaz EG. Hypothyroidism. Pediatr Rev 2014;35(8):336-47.

[25] Andrade CLO, Lemos AC, Machado GC, Fernandes LDC, Silva LL, Oliveira HB, et al. Congenital hypothyroidism as a risk factor for central hearing process disorders. Rev Paul Pediatr. 2019;37(1):82-9.

[26] Lorens A, Walkowiak A, Piotrowska A, Skarzynski H, Anderson I. ESRT and MCL correlations in experienced paediatric cochlear implant users. Cochlear Implants Int 2004;5(1):28-37.

[27] Raghunandhan S, Ravikumar A, Kameswaran M, Mandke K, Ranjith R. A clinical study of electrophysiological correlates of behavioural comfort levels in cochlear implantees. Cochlear Implants Int 2014;15(3):145-60.

Chapter 19

Treatment options for a baby with Luc's abscess

Mohamad N Salleh[1], MD
Mohd N Zakaria[2], PhD
and Nik AN Othman[1], MMed
[1]Department of Otorhinolaryngology Head and Neck Surgery, School of Medical Sciences, Universiti Sains Malaysia, Kelantan, Malaysia
[2]Audiology Programme, School of Health Sciences, Universiti Sains Malaysia, Kelantan, Malaysia

Abstract

Acute otitis media, an inflammation of the middle ear that causes hearing loss, occurs frequently in children. The complications of otitis media can be extracranial, intratemporal and intracranial. Luc's abscess is one of the extracranial complications that requires appropriate and timely treatment. In this chapter, we describe a challenging case of a 10-month-old boy with history of a recurrent posterior auricular subperiosteal abscess involving the mastoid bone with its clinical presentations, interesting images, and treatment options. The clinical management of Luc's abscess requires both medical and surgical considerations. High-resolution computed tomography (HRCT) findings are notably useful in the decision to perform mastoidectomy in uncertain cases.

Introduction

There are three types of hearing loss, i.e., conductive hearing loss (CHL), sensorineural hearing loss (SNHL) and mixed hearing loss (MHL) (1, 2).

In: Public Health: Audiology Research in Malaysia
Editors: Mohd N. Zakaria and Joav Merrick
ISBN: 979-8-89530-577-5

Acute otitis media (AOM), the presence of fluid in the middle ear, is a very common entity in childhood (3-5). It is also the main contributor to CHL among children (3). Acute mastoiditis may occur as an extension of the AOM. It rarely progresses to complications due to the advancements in modern antibiotics. However, complications are rising due to growing antibiotic resistance and an increasing number of immunocompromised patients leading to significant morbidity and mortality (6). Complications of otitis media are well known to be categorized into intratemporal, extracranial and intracranial complications (7). Extracranial consequences of otitis media are referred to as subperiosteal abscesses based on where they occur. Firstly coined by Henry Luc in 1913, Bezold's abscess and Citelli's abscess are infections that spread deeply to the sternocleidomastoid muscle and the digastric triangle, respectively. While the collection in Luc's abscess is situated beneath the temporal muscle. Its typical symptoms include swelling over the temporal or zygomatic region, associated with fever and ear pain (8). In this chapter, we report a challenging case highlighting the success of treatment options in a baby with Luc's abscess.

Case report

The case reported in this chapter was described based on the CARE guidelines (9), and the respective informed consent was obtained from the parent. In particular, a 10-month-old boy brought by his mother to the Otorhinolaryngology (ORL) Clinic, University Hospital presented with painful left posterosuperior auricular swelling for the past week. The swelling occurred at the sudden onset with a gradual increase in size. The mother also noted there was some collection inside the swelling area. The boy also had a fever for the past few days. Otherwise, the mother denied any insect bite before that, no trauma, no ear discharge, no facial asymmetry, no nasal symptoms, and was still active at home and tolerating feeding well. Additionally, the mother reported that her boy has a history of a similar presentation last two months and was admitted to another hospital, treated with an intravenous antibiotic for five days, and discharged home well without any surgical intervention.

Upon the examination, the boy was very active, not in septic looking, and afebrile. There was swelling at the left posterosuperior aspect about 5cm x 4 cm, soft in consistency, fluctuant, tender upon palpation, and no punctum or discharge with an inflamed surrounding area. The swelling pushed the left ear pinna inferiorly (Figure 1). On the otoscopy, the left tympanic membrane appeared inflamed, but no discharge was seen, while the opposite ear showed normal findings. Other than that, all other examinations were unremarkable.

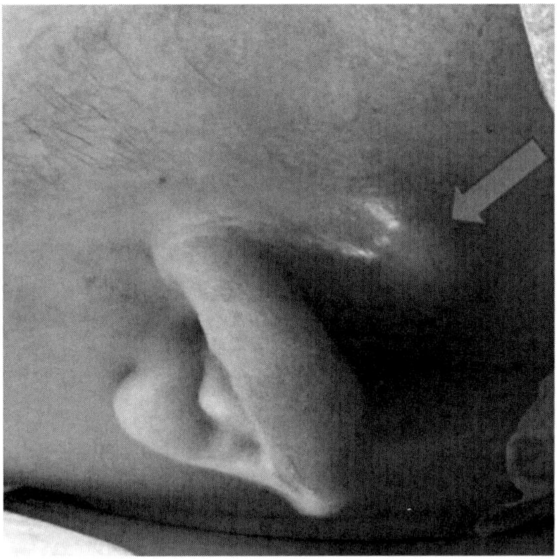

Figure 1. Swelling at the left posterosuperior part (as shown by the blue arrow) in which the ear pinna is pushed inferiorly with collection seen within the swelling.

The laboratory investigation showed significant increases in white blood cells, erythrocyte sedimentation rate (ESR), and c-reactive protein (CRP), indicating ongoing acute infection. The boy was then admitted to our ward and started on intravenous antibiotics, cefuroxime, and metronidazole. This boy also underwent high-resolution computed tomography (HRCT) to look for the origin and extension of the disease. As shown in Figure 2, the HRCT showed irregular rim enhancing heterogeneous hypodense collection at the left posterior auricular region measuring approximately 5.0 x 3.1 x 4.4 cm, with evidence of bony erosion of the mastoid air cells. The collection extends superiorly to the left temporalis muscle, which seems bulkier than the contralateral side. The collection pushes the left pinna inferiorly. The collection extends inferiorly to the lateral aspect of the left parotid gland. The left parotid gland appears bulky compared to the contralateral side; however, there is a clear plane between the collection and the left parotid gland (Figure 2).

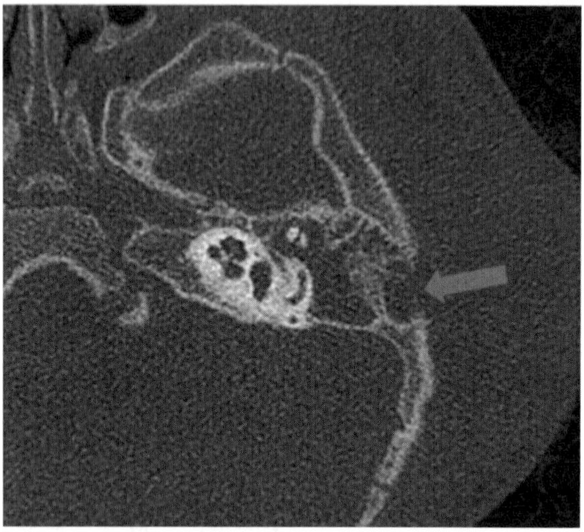

Figure 2. The HRCT temporal indicates hypodense collection at the left posterior auricular region and evidence of bony erosion of the mastoid air cells.

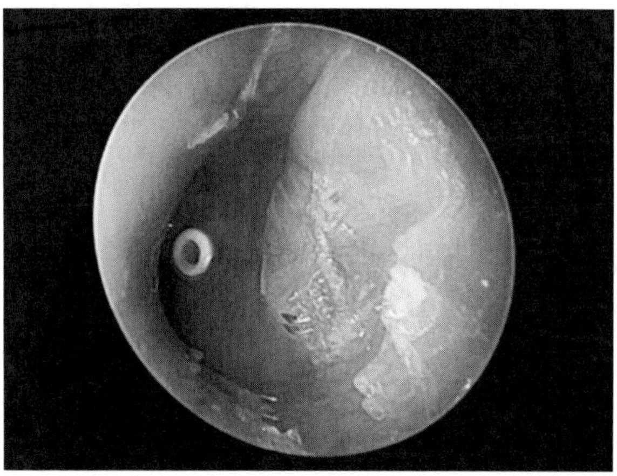

Figure 3. Myringotomy and grommet insertion are carried out, and mucous from the middle ear is drained out.

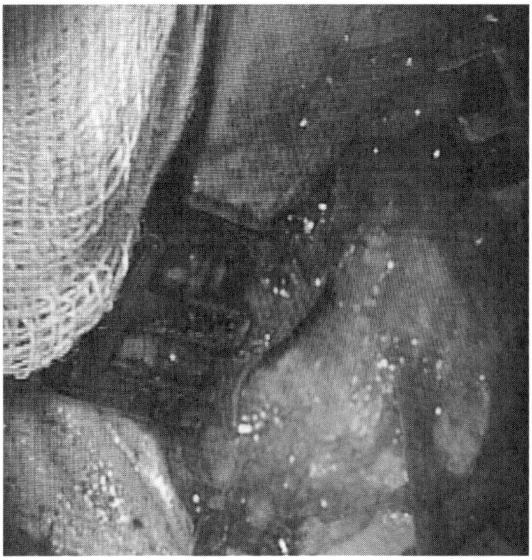

Figure 4. The cortical mastoidectomy procedure to clear the disease.

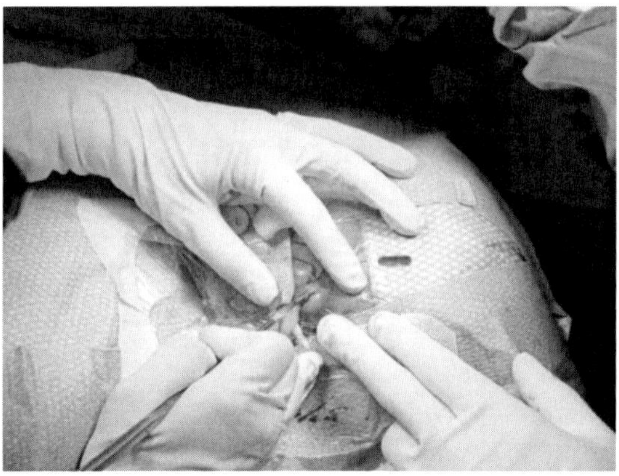

Figure 5. An incision is performed at the swelling site over the posterosuperior part of the ear pinna showing a lot of pus is drained out.

After 48 hours of the trial of antibiotics with slight improvement, this boy underwent left myringotomy grommet insertion, incision, and drainage of the left posterosuperior auricular swelling and followed by cortical mastoidectomy (Figures 3 and 4). During the procedure, lots of pus was drained out (Figure 5). Postoperatively, the baby responded well to the treatment and subsequently was discharged home without any complications.

Discussion

The management of acute mastoiditis complicated by a subperiosteal abscess traditionally requires mastoidectomy irrespective of the patient's age. With the improvement of antibiotic therapy, treating uncomplicated acute mastoiditis with myringotomy and intravenous antibiotic treatment might be beneficial (6).

In this chapter, the patient presented with left posterosuperior auricular swelling for the past weeks, followed by fever. He was subsequently admitted and started with a broad-spectrum antibiotic and HRCT of the temporal bone was performed as the preferred imaging modality. The reasons for the HRCT of the temporal bone are to exclude intracranial and extracranial complications, to confirm our diagnosis, and to determine the extension of the disease and status of the mastoid. The HRCT scan is notably useful in the decision making of either performing mastoidectomy or local drainage only.

The HRCT of the temporal bone uniquely features soft tissue density in the middle ear and mastoid cavity, erosion, or defect of cortical bone of the mastoid cavity, and contrast-enhanced subperiosteal shadows. In some cases, magnetic resonance imaging (MRI) may be necessary to determine intracranial complications (10). In cases of coalescent mastoiditis or cortical erosion of the mastoid, cortical mastoidectomy is recommended, especially in children after 48 hours of intravenous empirical antibiotics without signs of improvement (10). Treating Luc's abscess is best managed by a surgical approach. Abscess drainage, myringotomy (with or without grommet insertion), and cortical mastoidectomy were the favored surgeries in Luc's abscess. On the other hand, it is of utmost importance to empirically cover suspected Luc's abscess patients with broad spectrum intravenous antibiotics without waiting for culture and sensitivity tests.

Conclusion

Despite the increasingly effective antibiotic treatments, acute mastoiditis is still a worrying disease that seems to be growing in the pediatric age due to ever-increasing antibiotic resistance. Thorough history taking might be difficult in the pediatric age group; however, complete clinical examination is mandatory to avoid delays in diagnosis that can increase morbidity and mortality rates. The HRCT scan should be the investigation of choice to obtain a definitive diagnosis, identify associated mastoiditis, and rule out the possibility of intracranial complications. The HRCT findings will also help in the decision to perform mastoidectomy in uncertain cases. Cortical mastoidectomy is proven more effective than abscess drainage, especially in non-responding cases, extension into the mastoid bone, and paediatric patients.

Declaration of patient consent

The authors certify that they have obtained the consent form from the patient/guardian. In the form, the patient/guardian has given his/her consent for his/her image and other clinical information to be reported in the journal. The patient/guardian understands that his/her name and initial will not be published, and due efforts will be made to conceal his/her identity, but anonymity cannot be guaranteed.

References

[1] Lih AC, Zakaria MN, Mohamad RA, Nor Rashid MF. Effects of ethnicity and gender on the middle ear function in Asian adults. Indian J Otol 2017;23(2):94-7.

[2] Romli M, Wan Mohamad WN, Awang MA, Aw CL, Zakaria MN. The clinical value of bilateral bone conduction testing in hearing diagnosis. Indian J Otol 2020;26(3):182-5.

[3] Leung AKC, Wong AHC. Acute otitis media in children. Recent Pat Inflamm Allergy Drug Discov 2017;11:32-40.

[4] Dickson G. Acute otitis media. Prim Care 2014;41:11-8.

[5] Md Daud MK, Kamarulzaman N, Rahman NA, Zakaria MN. Sensorineural hearing loss in chronic suppurative otitis media. Int Med J 2013;20:559-60.

[6] Dagan R. Antibiotics for acute otitis media in the era of antibiotic resistance-what are the choices? Adv Exp Med Biol 2004;549:41-5.

[7] Thorne MC, Chewaproug L, Elden LM. Suppurative complications of acute otitis media. Arch Otolaryngol Head Neck Surg 2009;135:638-41.

[8] Fernandez IJ, Crocetta FM, Pelligra I, Burgio L, Demattè M. Clinical features and management of Luc's abscess: Case report and systematic review of the literature. Auris Nasus Larynx 2020;47:173-80.

[9] Gagnier JJ, Kienle G, Altman DG, Moher D, Sox H, Riley D; CARE Group. The CARE guidelines: consensus-based clinical case report guideline development. J Clin Epidemiol 2014;67:46-51.

[10] Kim SR, Choo OS, Park HY. Two cases of acute mastoiditis with subperiosteal abscess. Korean J Audiol 2013;17:97-100.

Chapter 20

Diagnosing Meniere's disease with pure tone audiometry

Mohd N Zakaria[1], PhD
Wan NW Mohamad[1], PhD
Cheu L Aw[1], MClinAud
Mohd FN Rashid[1], PhD
Mahamad A Awang[1], MClinAud
and Marniza Omar[2], PhD
[1]Audiology Programme, School of Health Sciences, Universiti Sains Malaysia, Kelantan, Malaysia
[2]Audiology Programme, Centre for Rehabilitation & Special Needs Studies, Faculty of Health Sciences, Universiti Kebangsaan Malaysia, Kuala Lumpur, Malaysia

Abstract

Meniere's disease is a chronic disorder of the inner ear that affects the balance and hearing of adult patients. To properly diagnose this ear problem, thorough history taking, otological examinations, and audiological assessments are needed. Having a specific indicator on an audiogram, i.e., low- to mid-frequency sensorineural hearing loss (SNHL), is essential to confirm the diagnosis of Meniere's disease. However, there is a lack of clarity regarding the specific frequencies, particularly those related to bone conduction (BC) thresholds on the audiogram, that should be taken into account for the purpose of establishing the diagnosis. This chapter emphasizes the significance of incorporating the 250 Hz BC threshold in the evaluation of a patient with Meniere's disease. While there may be debate surrounding the

In: Public Health: Audiology Research in Malaysia
Editors: Mohd N. Zakaria and Joav Merrick
ISBN: 979-8-89530-577-5

measurement of this threshold, the case report presented illustrates the value of including it in order to make an accurate diagnosis.

Introduction

Maintaining healthy hearing is essential for effective communication and participation in daily activities (1). If the hearing mechanism is compromised, it can lead to hearing loss and related symptoms (2-6). There are three main types of hearing loss: conductive hearing loss (CHL), sensorineural hearing loss (SNHL), and mixed hearing loss (MHL) (1). The severity of hearing loss can range from mild to profound. The CHL is typically caused by problems affecting the tympanic membrane, middle ear, or external ear canal (7). On the other hand, the SNHL occurs when the inner ear or neural part of the hearing system is impaired (1). The MHL is a condition where both CHL and SNHL are present. Treatment options vary, with SNHL often managed with hearing aids and CHL typically addressed through medication or surgery (1).

In clinical settings, hearing diagnosis is typically made by means of pure tone audiometry (PTA) (1, 2). In this testing, air conduction (AC) and bone conduction (BC) thresholds are determined at specific frequencies (2). Displayed on an audiogram, the AC and BC thresholds are used to indicate the severity of hearing loss and the type of hearing loss, respectively (1). In CHL cases, while the BC thresholds are within the normal range ($\leq$ 20 dB HL), the AC thresholds are abnormal (exceeding 20 dB HL), and significant air-bone gaps (ABGs) are noted. In contrast, those with SNHL will show abnormal AC and BC thresholds (with no ABGs). Meanwhile, in MHL cases, significant ABGs are present, and both AC and BC thresholds are outside the normal range.

Meniere's disease is one of the otological conditions that can cause SNHL (1, 8). It is a chronic disorder of the inner ear that affects balance and hearing. The primary symptoms of Meniere's disease are recurrent, spontaneous episodes of vertigo or dizziness, hearing loss, tinnitus, and a sensation of fullness or pressure in the ear (8). The onset of symptoms is often unpredictable and can last from twenty minutes to several hours. The severity of symptoms varies from person to person, with some experiencing mild episodes of imbalance, while others suffer severe vertigo that can lead to falls or drop attacks. The exact cause of Meniere's disease is not fully understood. Nevertheless, it is believed to be related to an abnormality in the volume or composition of the fluid in the inner ear, known as endolymph. Factors that may contribute to this abnormality include improper fluid drainage due to blockages or anatomical abnormalities, immune system response, viral infections, and genetic predispositions (8).

In clinical practice, patients with suspected Meniere's disease will undergo comprehensive history taking, otological assessments, and audiological evaluations (1). Apart from the typical complaints (episodic vertigo, fluctuating hearing loss, aural fullness, and tinnitus), having audiogram results (indicating low- to mid-frequency SNHL) is one of the strong indicators for diagnosing Meniere's disease, as outlined by the American Academy of Otolaryngology-Head and Neck Surgery (AAO-HNS) (9, 10). Nevertheless, it is unclear which frequencies (on the audiogram, particularly BC thresholds) should be considered in order to make the diagnosis. It is worth stating that some studies considered 500 Hz as the lowest frequency when assessing the hearing status of their subjects with Meniere's disease (11, 12). In this chapter, the importance of including the BC threshold at 250 Hz when assessing a patient with Meniere's disease is highlighted.

Case report

This is a case involving a 55-year-old Malay man who was referred by an otorhinolaryngology (ORL) specialist for comprehensive audiological assessments. He had noticed a decrease in hearing in his left ear approximately four months ago, with fluctuations in his hearing ability. Additionally, he mentioned experiencing a high-pitched ringing sound in the same ear, which worsened in quiet environments or when his ear was blocked. Despite this, the tinnitus did not significantly impact his daily life activities or sleep. Over the past month, he also reported feeling fullness in his ear and episodes of dizziness lasting 2-3 days per attack, with three attacks so far. The man had previously worked in construction, where he was exposed to loud noises from using a jackhammer for about a year. He also has a history of hypertension and allergic rhinitis, for which he was on continuous medications. There were no reported instances of otalgia, otorrhea, or other ear-related conditions.

On today's visit, the otoscopic examination revealed unremarkable findings bilaterally. He then underwent the tympanometry, acoustic reflex, and PTA assessments, based on the recommended test protocols (13-15). For this purpose, a 226 Hz tympanometer (GSI TympStar Pro, Grason-Stadler Inc., USA) was used. As revealed, he was found to have normal middle ear function (i.e., type A tympanogram for each ear). He also elicited normal acoustic reflex thresholds ipsilaterally (i.e., 70-100 dB) at 500 Hz, 1000 Hz, and 2000 Hz frequencies. Using a two-channel audiometer (GSI 61, Grason-Stadler Inc., USA), his hearing status was assessed. The AC and BC thresholds were determined using the TDH-39 headphone and the B71 bone vibrator, respectively. The audiogram in Figure 1 displays the results for both ears. As illustrated, the right ear showed normal hearing, but the left ear exhibited mild hearing loss at specific frequencies including 250 Hz, 3000 Hz, 4000 Hz, and 6000 Hz, while other frequencies were within the normal range. By considering the BC thresholds (particularly at 250 Hz), the type of hearing loss for the left ear was likely to be SNHL.

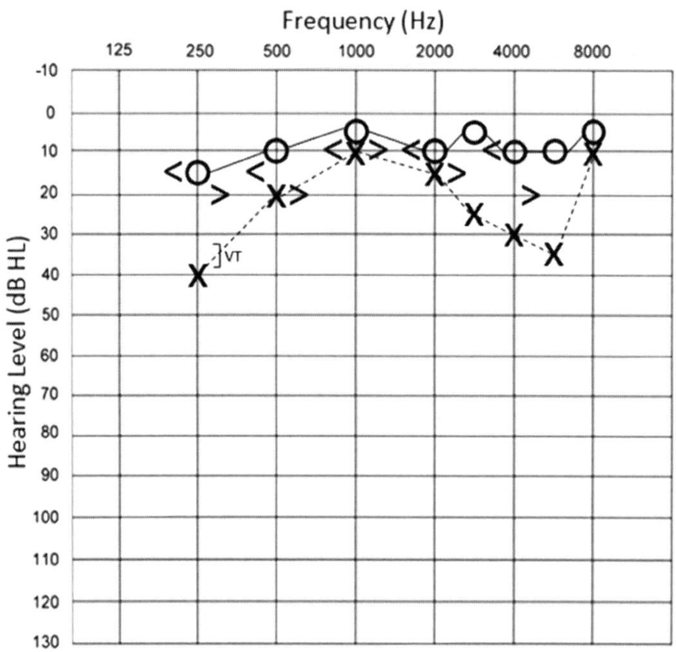

Figure 1. Pure tone audiometry (PTA) results of the patient.

Discussion

To assist in the proper diagnosis of patients with Meniere's disease, the AAO-HNS has produced specific guidelines (with four categories, i.e., "certain," "definite," "possible," and "probable" Meniere's disease) (9, 10). Based on his symptoms and audiological results, the patient in this case report is likely to fall under the "definite" Meniere's disease category.

Nevertheless, his audiometric results necessitate additional consideration. The AC and BC thresholds were documented at many frequencies, including at 250 Hz. For his left ear, a clear indicator supporting the diagnosis of SNHL was only evident at 250 Hz. At this frequency, both AC and BC thresholds exceeded the normal range, with no significant ABG present. Whereas at 500 Hz and 1000 Hz, the AC and BC thresholds were within the normal limits. In this regard, if the BC threshold was not assessed at 250 Hz, it would be problematic to confirm the type of hearing loss (as well as for Meniere's disease diagnosis). While tympanometry and acoustic reflex test results may indicate no CHL, it is still important to confirm this with information from the audiogram.

It is worth mentioning that some clinical centres do not recommend the measurement of the BC threshold at 250 Hz (16), due to the design and limitations of the bone vibrator. Specifically, the conventional B71 bone vibrator may produce questionable ABGs resulting from vibrotactile responses and harmonic distortions in normal-hearing individuals and those with SNHL (17-19). In this regard, the occurrence of significant ABGs could be erroneously associated with the presence of CHL instead of SNHL (which could lead to misdiagnosis). Additionally, patients with Meniere's disease have been found to have large ABGs at lower frequencies, particularly with the 250 Hz frequency showing the most pronounced ABGs (20, 21). This finding would further "diminish" the usefulness of BC thresholds in such cases. Instead of being attributed to technical problems with bone vibrators, factors such as increased endolymphatic pressure reducing stapes mobility and reduced stapedial mobility due to saccular dilatation exerting pressure on the stapedial footplate have been suggested as reasons for the significant ABGs observed in Meniere's disease cases (20, 22). Nonetheless, as demonstrated in this case report, having the BC threshold at 250 Hz is indeed useful and provides a sensible result for hearing diagnosis in the left ear (as well as aiding in confirming the diagnosis of Meniere's disease). The presence of mild hearing loss at high frequencies (with a notch at 6 kHz for the BC threshold) is consistent with the patient's reported exposure to loud noises.

In the context of case management, the patient's hearing will be monitored on a regular basis. He was referred back to the ORL specialist to address his symptoms and is to be treated as a case of Meniere's disease.

Conclusion

Patients who are suspected to have Meniere's disease need to undergo a thorough diagnosis process. In addition to documenting the typical symptoms of this chronic inner ear problem, obtaining accurate audiometric results is crucial for confirming the diagnosis. Herein, it is advisable to measure the AC and BC thresholds at various frequencies, including at 250 Hz, despite the technical issues that may impact the accuracy of the BC threshold at that frequency.

Declaration of patient consent

The authors certify that they have obtained the consent form from the patient. In the form, the patient has given his consent for his image and other clinical information to be reported in the journal. The patient understands that his name and initial will not be published, and due efforts will be made to conceal his identity, but anonymity cannot be guaranteed.

References

[1] Katz J, Marshall C, English K, Hood L, Tillery KL. Handbook of clinical audiology. Philadelphia: Lippincott Williams Wilkins, 2015.

[2] Wan Mohamad WN, Romli M, Awang MA, Abdullah R, Lih AC, Zakaria MN. The presence of unusual bone conduction thresholds in pure tone audiometry. Indian J Otol 2020;26(1):54-7.

[3] Zainun Z, Zakaria MN, Sidek D, Ismail Z. Clinical use of Malay version of vertigo symptom scale (MVSS) in patients with peripheral vestibular disorder (PVD). Med J Malaysia 2012;67(4):386-9.

[4] Wong JW, Wan Mohamad WN, Wan Husain WS, Zakaria MN. The tinnitus suppressive effect: Comparisons between three types of maskers. Int J Disabil Hum Dev 2020;19(1):21-6.

[5] Zakaria MN. The effectiveness of sound therapy in treating patients with mild and severe tinnitus. Int J Disabil Hum Dev 2020;19(2):215-9.

[6] Abdul Wahab NA, Wahab S, Abdul Rahman AH, Sidek D, Zakaria MN. The hyperactivity of efferent auditory system in patients with schizophrenia: a transient evoked otoacoustic emissions study. Psychiatry Investig 2016;13(1):82-8.

[7] Zakaria MN, Romli M, Mohamad WNW, Awang MA, Wahab NAA. The diagnostic value of tympanometric width in identifying middle ear disorders. Indian J Otol 2020;26(3):186-90.

[8] Gibson WPR. Meniere's Disease. Adv Otorhinolaryngol 2019;82:77-86.

[9] Goebel JA. 2015 Equilibrium Committee amendment to the 1995 AAO-HNS guidelines for the definition of Ménière's disease. Otolaryngol Head Neck Surg 2016;154(3):403-4.

[10] Lopez-Escamez JA, Carey J, Chung WH, Goebel JA, Magnusson M, Mandalà M, et al. Diagnostic criteria for Menière's disease. J Vestib Res 2015;25(1):1-7.

[11] Yetişer S, Kertmen M. Cochlear conductive hearing loss in patients with Meniere's disease. Kulak Burun Bogaz Ihtis Derg 2007;17(1):18-21.

[12] Pai I, Connor S. Low frequency air-bone gap in Meniere's disease: relationship with magnetic resonance imaging features of endolymphatic hydrops. Ear Hear 2022;43(6):1678-86.

[13] Romli M, Wan Mohamad WN, Awang MA, Aw CL, Zakaria MN. The clinical value of bilateral bone conduction testing in hearing diagnosis. Indian J Otol 2020;26(3):182-5.

[14] Lih AC, Zakaria MN, Mohamad RA, Nor Rashid MF. Effects of ethnicity and gender on the middle ear function in Asian adults. Indian J Otol 2017;23(2):94-7.

[15] Awang MA, Zakaria MN. Acoustic reflex testing in clinical audiology: What is the next direction? Int J Disabil Hum Dev 2019;18(2):123-8.

[16] Manual for Audiology Clinical Educators 2018: The University of Melbourne. URL: https://healthsciences.unimelb.edu.au/__data/assets/pdf_file/0011/2650709/Clinical-Educator-Manual-2018.pdf.

[17] Eichenauer A, Dillon H, Clinch B, Loi T. Effect of bone-conduction harmonic distortions on hearing thresholds. J Acoust Soc Am 2014;136(2):EL96-102.

[18] Fröhlich L, Plontke SK, Rahne T. Influence of transducer types on bone conduction hearing thresholds. PLoS One 2018;13:e0195233.

[19] Jansson KJ, Håkansson B, Johannsen L, Tengstrand T. Electro-acoustic performance of the new bone vibrator radioear B81: A comparison with the conventional radioear B71. Int J Audiol 2015;54:334-40.

[20] Lee HJ, Jeon JH, Park S, Kim BG, Lee WS, Kim SH. Prevalence and clinical significance of spontaneous low-frequency air-bone gaps in Ménière's disease. Otol Neurotol 2014;35(3):489-94.

[21] Sugimoto S, Yoshida T, Teranishi M, Okazaki Y, Naganawa S, Sone M. The relationship between endolymphatic hydrops in the vestibule and low-frequency air-bone gaps. Laryngoscope 2018;128(7):1658-62.

[22] Muchnik C, Hildesheimer M, Rubinstein M, Arenberg IK. Low frequency air-bone gap in Meniere's disease without middle ear pathology. A preliminary report. Am J Otol 1989;10:1-4.

Chapter 21

The audiometric Weber test versus the tuning fork Weber test for hearing diagnosis: Which one is better?

Mohd N Zakaria, PhD
Audiology Programme, School of Health Sciences, Universiti Sains Malaysia, Kelantan, Malaysia

Abstract

In clinical settings, hearing impairment is typically diagnosed using pure tone audiometry (PTA). By determining air conduction (AC) and bone conduction (BC) thresholds, the severity of hearing loss and the type of hearing loss for each ear can be documented. Nevertheless, the PTA outcomes can be questionable in some cases, in which the results from other tests are required to verify the hearing diagnosis. In this chapter reporting a 32-year-old man diagnosed with a mild traumatic brain injury, the clinical usefulness of performing the audiometric Weber test for confirming the type of hearing loss is highlighted. Herein, PTA, tympanometry and tuning fork Rinne test yielded contradictory results, and the tuning fork Weber test was unsuccessful. As such, the incorporation of the audiometric Weber test into the routine audiological evaluation protocol can be beneficial to achieve an accurate hearing diagnosis.

Introduction

The sense of hearing plays a crucial role in facilitating daily activities and communication. Any impairment or damage to the hearing organs can lead to

In: Public Health: Audiology Research in Malaysia
Editors: Mohd N. Zakaria and Joav Merrick
ISBN: 979-8-89530-577-5

hearing loss and associated symptoms (1-5). In clinical settings, specialized audiological assessments are utilized to accurately diagnose hearing impairment (6-11). Herein, pure tone audiometry (PTA) is widely recognized as the primary diagnostic test for assessing hearing abilities (1, 12). Through the measurement of air conduction (AC) and bone conduction (BC) thresholds, this test enables the determination of the degree and type of hearing loss. The degree of hearing loss varies from mild to profound, and there are three types of hearing loss: conductive hearing loss (where the external and middle ears are affected), sensorineural hearing loss (that occurs when the inner ear and/or auditory nerve are compromised), and mixed hearing loss (a combination of conductive hearing loss and sensorineural hearing loss) (12). Upon establishing the hearing diagnosis, timely initiation of appropriate treatment and/or intervention can be implemented to mitigate the adverse effects of hearing impairment.

It is worth stating that the tuning fork tests, including the Rinne and Weber tests, continue to be commonly utilized by otorhinolaryngology (ORL) specialists for the purpose of determining the type of hearing loss (13, 14). In the Weber test, the tester holds a low-frequency tuning fork (either 256 or 512 Hz) by its stem and struck one of its prongs against his/her elbow at the upper one-third end. Then, the stem of the resonating tuning fork was firmly placed in the midline of the forehead. In cases of normal hearing, a central perception is expected (14). On the other hand, patients with unilateral conductive hearing loss will report the tone lateralized to the affected ear. Whereas for those with unilateral sensorineural hearing loss, the tone will be heard louder in the normal ear (14). It is essential to note that the sensitivity and specificity of the Weber test for hearing diagnosis are reasonably high (15, 16).

The Weber test can also be conducted using the standard audiometer, referred to as an audiometric Weber test, which offers similar efficacy in identifying the type of hearing loss along with additional advantages (14). Nevertheless, conducting more studies is beneficial to further verify the importance of this test for hearing diagnosis. As such, the case reported in this chapter aimed to highlight the clinical usefulness of performing the audiometric Weber test as a means of corroborating the hearing diagnosis when discrepancies were observed across the tests (as well as when the tuning fork Weber test was not informative).

Case report

A 32-year-old man, diagnosed with a mild traumatic brain injury resulting from a motor vehicle accident (MVA), was referred by an ORL specialist for comprehensive audiological assessments. The patient reported reduced hearing bilaterally, with a more pronounced loss in the left ear following the MVA. The CT scan of the brain revealed a subdural hematoma in the right frontoparietal area and a subarachnoid haemorrhage in the right frontal and temporal regions. Additionally, a bone fracture was noted in the left parietotemporal area. The patient also experienced dizziness, particularly when lying down, which lasted for a few seconds. No other significant findings were obtained during the history taking.

All audiological assessments were conducted in a dedicated soundproof room within the Audiology Clinic, University Hospital. The otoscopic examination revealed an intact tympanic membrane and a clear ear canal for each ear. The PTA testing was carried out based on the recommended protocol and a two-channel audiometer (GSI 61, Grason-Stadler Inc., USA) was used for this purpose. The TDH-39 headphone and B71 bone vibrator were employed to determine the respective AC and BC thresholds. As shown in Figure 1, he was found to have a mild sensorineural hearing loss in the right ear. In his left ear, a mild to moderate sensorineural hearing loss was noted. On the other hand, by using a 226 Hz tympanometer (GSI TympStar Pro, Grason-Stadler Inc, USA), a type B tympanogram was obtained for each ear, suggesting the presence of conductive pathology in the middle ear. Herein, the PTA and tympanometric results were not consistent with each other, and an additional assessment should be conducted to verify the exact type of hearing loss. It is worth mentioning that the tuning fork Rinne test (that was carried out by the ORL specialist on the same day with the audiological assessments) revealed a positive Rinne result for each ear (indicating the absence of conductive pathology bilaterally). The tuning fork Weber test was attempted, but the patient was not able to perceive the bone-conducted tone appropriately (as the test room was reasonably noisy). In view of this, an audiometric Weber test was conducted at frequencies of 250 Hz and 500 Hz. This test was performed based on the method suggested by Abdullah et al. (14). In particular, the B71 bone vibrator was placed at the midline of the forehead and the tone was presented at 20 dB sensation level (i.e., 20 dB above the hearing threshold of the test frequency). The patient was then instructed to report whether the tone was heard louder in either ear or equally loud (i.e., central perception). For both frequencies tested, the tones were clearly perceived in the right ear, indicating the absence of conductive pathology in the left ear (or better BC thresholds in the right ear). This result is indeed consistent with the PTA and Rinne test outcomes. The type of hearing loss was concluded to be sensorineural hearing loss for both ears.

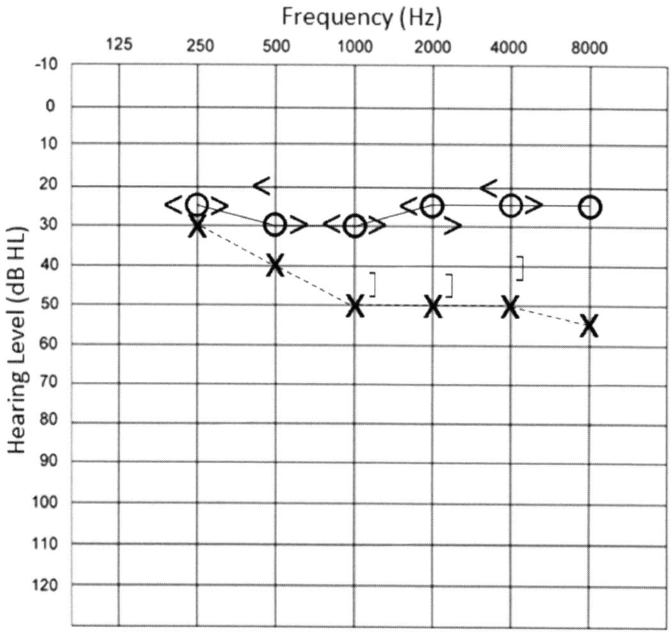

Figure 1. Pure tone audiometry (PTA) results of the patient.

Discussion

While the PTA testing is frequently utilized for assessing the severity and type of hearing loss, it is important to note that there are certain limitations associated with its use (1, 18). In cases where discrepancies arise among the test results, additional evaluations should be undertaken to reach a definitive determination of the hearing diagnosis. It is essential to accurately diagnose hearing loss in order to effectively apply specific treatment approaches.

In this chapter, the patient was diagnosed to have a mild sensorineural hearing loss at high frequencies in each ear. This result, nevertheless, was not consistent with that of tympanometry. According to the tympanometric finding, both middle ears were abnormal (possibly filled with fluid), and conductive hearing loss should be present. However, the audiogram did not show any significant air-bone gaps, indicating that the type of hearing loss was likely sensorineural rather than conductive in nature. In light of this, the audiometric Weber test was performed, and the finding confirmed that the type of hearing loss in both ears was indeed sensorineural. Recall that in this test, the patient perceived the tones as being louder in the right ear, indicating sound lateralization towards the right ear. This response implied the absence of conductive hearing loss in the left ear, consistent with the PTA result. According to the findings of the Rinne test, PTA, and audiometric Weber test, the left ear also exhibited sensorineural hearing loss, contrary to the indication of conductive hearing loss based on the tympanometric result. Herein, given that the tympanometry did not achieve 100% specificity (18,19), it is therefore possible to suggest the existence of conductive pathology, despite the middle ear being deemed healthy.

To aid in the hearing diagnosis, the tuning fork Weber test was also carried out, but the patient failed to perceive the tone as the noise level in the room was reasonably high. Apart from the noisy room factor, there are other aspects known to affect the outcomes of this test (14). Among others, it is challenging to maintain a consistent force to the designated area, when the test is repeated. The tester must also be skilled and experienced to effectively administer the test. Moreover, tuning forks exhibit specific decay times that must be taken into consideration during the testing (i.e., the patient must give the response as soon as possible, while the tone is still audible) (20). The audiometric Weber test, on the other hand, presents several advantages over the tuning fork Weber test, such as the ability to control sound presentation at desired intensity levels (without decay issue), assess multiple frequencies, and provide a constant force to the surface area of the forehead (14).

In terms of the case management, the patient's hearing will be monitored from time to time. This is because most head injury cases will show hearing improvements over time (21). The patient was also reluctant to try or wear hearing aids, but he will consider this option in the future should his hearing condition deteriorate further. Additionally, due to his report of experiencing dizziness, the Dix-Hallpike test was performed, revealing a diagnosis of benign paroxysmal positional vertigo (BPPV) affecting his left posterior semicircular canal. Subsequently, the Epley maneuver was carried out, and it effectively resolved his BPPV problem. He will also need to attend sessions at the ORL clinic as scheduled.

Conclusion

The case reported in this chapteremphasizes the importance of conducting the audiometric Weber test when the results of other tests are inconsistent. Given its advantages, the inclusion of the audiometric Weber test into the routine audiological evaluation protocol can be advantageous to achieve an accurate hearing diagnosis.

Declaration of patient consent

The author certifies that he has obtained the consent form from the patient. In the form, the patient has given his consent for his image and other clinical information to be reported in the journal. The patient understands that his name and initial will not be published, and due efforts will be made to conceal his identity, but anonymity cannot be guaranteed.

References

[1] Wan Mohamad WN, Romli M, Awang MA, Abdullah R, Lih AC, Zakaria MN. The presence of unusual bone conduction thresholds in pure tone audiometry. Indian J Otol 2020;26(1):54-7.

[2] Zainun Z, Zakaria MN, Sidek D, Ismail Z. Clinical use of Malay version of vertigo symptom scale (MWSS) in patients with peripheral vestibular disorder (PVD). Med J Malaysia 2012;67(4):386-9.

[3] Wong JW, Wan Mohamad WN, Wan Husain WS, Zakaria MN. The tinnitus suppressive effect: Comparisons between three types of maskers. Int J Disabil Hum Dev 2020;19(1):21-6.

[4] Zakaria MN. The effectiveness of sound therapy in treating patients with mild and severe tinnitus. Int J Disabil Hum Dev 2020;19(2):215-9.

[5] Abdul Wahab NA, Wahab S, Abdul Rahman AH, Sidek D, Zakaria MN. The hyperactivity of efferent auditory system in patients with schizophrenia: a transient evoked otoacoustic emissions study. Psychiatry Investig 2016;13(1):82-8.

[6] Romli M, Wan Mohamad WN, Awang MA, Aw CL, Zakaria MN. The clinical value of bilateral bone conduction testing in hearing diagnosis. Indian J Otol 2020;26(3):182-5.

[7] Lih AC, Zakaria MN, Mohamad RA, Nor Rashid MF. Effects of ethnicity and gender on the middle ear function in Asian adults. Indian J Otol 2017;23(2):94-7.

[8] Abdul Wahid SN, Md Daud MK, Sidek D, Abd Rahman N, Mansor S, Zakaria MN. The performance of distortion product otoacoustic emissions and automated

auditory brainstem response in the same ear of the babies in neonatal unit. Int J Pediatr Otorhinolaryngol 2012;76(9):1366-9.

[9] Zakaria MN, Wahab NAA, Maamor N, Jalaei B, Dzulkarnain AAA. Auditory brainstem response (ABR) findings in males and females with comparable head sizes at supra-threshold and threshold levels. Neurol Psychiatry Brain Res 2019;32:4-7.

[10] Jalaei B, Azmi MHAM, Zakaria MN. Gender differences in binaural speech-evoked auditory brainstem response: are they clinically significant? Braz J Otorhinolaryngol 2019;85(4):486-93.

[11] Zakaria MN, Jalaei B, Wahab NA. Gender and modulation frequency effects on auditory steady state response (ASSR) thresholds. Eur Arch Otorhinolaryngol 2016;273(2):349-54.

[12] Katz J, Marshall C, English K, Hood L, Tillery KL, eds. Handbook of clinical audiology. Philadelphia, PA: Lippincott Williams Wilkins, 2015.

[13] Kelly EA, Li B, Adams ME. Diagnostic accuracy of tuning fork tests for hearing loss: a systematic review. Otolaryngol Head Neck Surg 2018;159(2):220-30.

[14] Abdullah SN, Zakaria MN, Salim R, Md Daud MK, Nik Othman NA. Comparing the diagnostic accuracy of audiometric Weber test and tuning fork Weber test in patients with conductive hearing loss. Laryngoscope Investig Otolaryngol 2022;7(2):523-9.

[15] Stankiewicz JA, Mowry HJ. Clinical accuracy of tuning fork tests. Laryngoscope 1979;89(12):1956-63.

[16] Shuman AG, Li X, Halpin CF, Rauch SD, Telian SA. Tuning fork testing in sudden sensorineural hearing loss. JAMA Intern Med 2013;173(8):706-7.

[17] Zakaria MN. The limitations of pure-tone audiometry (as the gold standard test of hearing) that are worthy of consideration. Indian J Otol 2021;27(1):1-2.

[18] Szucs E, Diependaele R, Clement PA. The accuracy of tympanometry assessed by its sensitivity and specificity. Acta Otorhinolaryngol Belg 1995;49(3):287-92.

[19] Rogers DJ, Boseley ME, Adams MT, Makowski RL, Hohman MH. Prospective comparison of handheld pneumatic otoscopy, binocular microscopy, and tympanometry in identifying middle ear effusions in children. Int J Pediatr Otorhinolaryngol 2010;74(10):1140-3.

[20] Miller GW. Tuning fork decay. Laryngoscope 1979;89(3):459-72.

[21] Podoshin L, Fradis M. Hearing loss after head injury. Arch Otolaryngol 1975;101(1):15-8.

Chapter 22

The clinical value of the subjective visual vertical (SVV) test with a complex visual image

Rosdan Salim[1], MMed
Nurul SM Sakeri[2], PhD
Saiful A Jamaluddin[2], PhD
Nor HA Wahat[3], PhD
and Mohd N Zakaria[4], PhD

[1]Department of Otorhinolaryngology, School of Medical Sciences, Universiti Sains Malaysia, Kelantan, Malaysia
[2]Department of Audiology and Speech-Language Pathology, Kuliyyah of Allied Health Sciences, International Islamic University Malaysia, Pahang, Malaysia
[3]Audiology Program, Centre for Rehabilitation & Special Needs Studies, Faculty of Health Sciences, Universiti Kebangsaan Malaysia, Kuala Lumpur, Malaysia
[4]Audiology Programme, School of Health Sciences, Universiti Sains Malaysia, Kelantan, Malaysia

Abstract

Comprehensive history taking and specialized vestibular assessments are required to appropriately diagnose patients with vestibular disorders. In line with the advancement in medical technology, more options are now available to assess and treat patients with vestibular symptoms in clinical settings. The subjective visual vertical (SVV) test is valuable to identify those with problems affecting the otolith organs. The SVV angle can be determined using simple or complex visual images. In this chapter reporting a 48-year-old lady with an imbalance problem, we demonstrate the importance of including the complex visual image in the SVV test in

In: Public Health: Audiology Research in Malaysia
Editors: Mohd N. Zakaria and Joav Merrick
ISBN: 979-8-89530-577-5

order to achieve an accurate vestibular diagnosis. While abnormal results were found in other vestibular tests, her SVV result was found to be within the normal limits for a simple solid line image. Nevertheless, an abnormal SVV angle was noted when an arrow pattern was used as the visual image. In conclusion, the SVV test employing a complex visual image appears to be a more effective method for identifying vestibular dysfunction.

Introduction

Maintaining a healthy balance function is crucial for performing daily tasks effectively. The balance system plays a vital role in controlling postural control, gait, and overall coordination of the body by integrating various sensory inputs from the visual, somatosensory, and vestibular systems (1). The vestibular organs, which include semicircular canals and otolith organs (saccule and utricle), have been preserved throughout evolution and perform a variety of functions. In particular, the semicircular canals detect rotational movements of the head, whereas the otolith organs detect linear movements in both vertical and horizontal planes, as well as head tilt and the influence of gravity (2).

Dizziness is a common symptom experienced by individuals with impaired vestibular functions (3). It can have a significant impact on an individual's quality of life, as the underlying cause can range from benign and self-limiting to severe and potentially life-threatening. Since there are various types of dizziness (e.g., vertigo, lightheadedness, pre-syncope, and disequilibrium), establishing an accurate diagnosis is therefore crucial so that appropriate treatment can be provided in a timely manner (3).

In line with the advancement in medical technology, more options are now available to properly evaluate vestibular functions in clinical settings (2). The status of semicircular canals can be conveniently assessed with videonystagmography (VNG), video head impulse test (vHIT), dynamic visual acuity (DVA) test, and others (4-6). On the other hand, cervical vestibular evoked myogenic potential (cVEMP), ocular vestibular evoked myogenic potential (oVEMP), subjective visual vertical (SVV) test, and subjective visual horizontal (SVH) test are among the specialized assessments to evaluate the function of otolith organs (7-12). Nevertheless, continual research endeavours have been undertaken to identify the most effective vestibular assessments and protocols. In a typical SVV test, an individual is seated and manipulates a laser projection line using a remote control to align it with his/her perceived vertical position. Using a solid line as the visual image, the deviation from the true vertical position (i.e., 0°) that is within ± 2° is considered normal (10, 11). However, when a complex visual image was used (such as an arrow pattern), larger SVV angles were noted among those with normal balance functions (i.e., up to 2.33°) (11). In view of this, it is uncertain if using a complex visual image in the SVV test would be more effective in detecting patients with utricular dysfunction. In this chapter, we demonstrate the importance of including the complex visual image in the SVV test in order to achieve an accurate vestibular diagnosis.

Case report

A 48-year-old woman, with the main complaint of imbalance, underwent comprehensive audiological assessments. The imbalance problem started about two months ago affecting her ability to pursue daily life activities. In particular, she felt imbalance while walking (and she had to walk slowly to avoid fall). Additionally, she experienced dizziness and nausea, particularly when driving her car. The dizziness also occurred when her head was moved quickly (and she would avoid quick head movements whenever necessary). She also noticed some difficulties to understand conversations, especially in noisy situations. She did not experience otalgia, otorrhea or other otological diseases. No other significant findings were obtained in the history taking.

To assess her vestibular functions, several assessments were conducted. To quantify the severity of the problem, the Malay version of vertigo symptom scale (MVVSS) questionnaire was administered (3). The score was reasonably high (i.e., 31), consistent with her self-reported symptoms. In the Fukuda stepping test, an angle rotation of about 50° (to the right side) was noted. On the other hand, unremarkable findings were obtained in the Dix-Hallpike, side lying and supine roll tests, suggesting the absence of a vestibular pathology such as benign paroxysmal positional vertigo (BPPV). To assess the vestibulo-ocular reflex (VOR) of the patient, the vHIT was conducted based on the recommended procedure (5). Employing the Synapsys® vHIT Ulmer system (Marseilles, France), her VOR gain values (ranging from 0.83 to 1.08) were found to be within the normal limits for all canals tested. The oculomotor tests (saccade and smooth pursuit) also revealed normal findings.

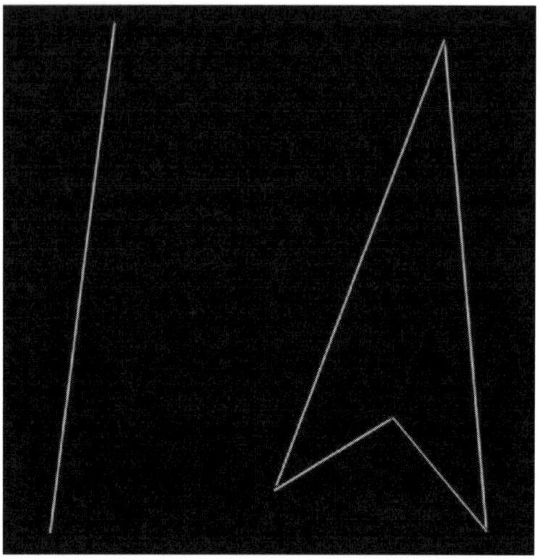

Figure 1. Computerized visual images (solid line and arrow pattern) used in the subjective visual vertical test.

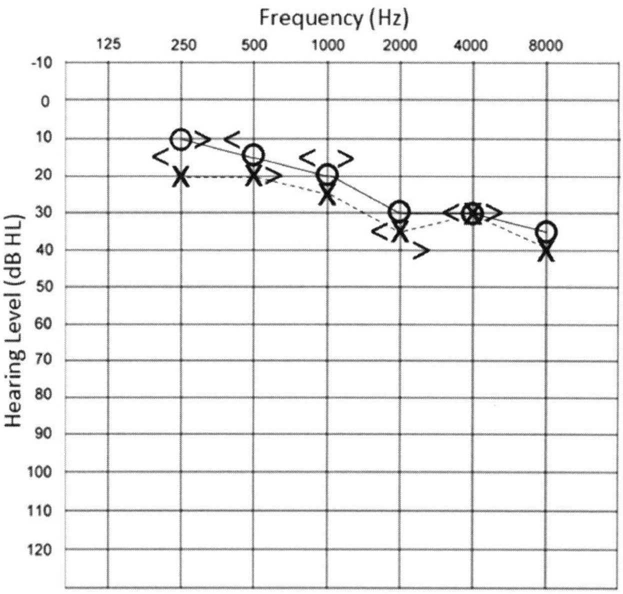

Figure 2. Pure tone audiometry (PTA) results of the patient.

To evaluate the function of the otolith organs, air-conducted cVEMP and oVEMP assessments were carried out according to the recommended protocols (8,9). The Eclipse EP25 device (Interacoustics, Assens, Denmark) was used for both tests, and a 500 Hz tone burst was chosen as the stimulus. In the cVEMP testing, a clear cVEMP response was observed for each ear (with an interaural amplitude ratio of 13.8%). However, while a good oVEMP waveform was noted in the left ear, no identifiable peaks were observed in the right ear (implying a right utricular dysfunction). To verify these findings, the computerized SVV system (version 1.3.0 by Synapsys, Marseille, France) was employed to determine the verticality perception based on the suggested method (11). In this assessment, two different visual images were used, i.e., solid line and arrow pattern (Figure 1). The patient was seated in an upright position on a designated chair and instructed to wear a vision field mask to eliminate visual cues. She was then tasked with aligning a visual image vertically using the provided control joystick. It was found that her ability to perceive the verticality of the solid line image seemed to be unaffected (i.e., SVV angle of 1.7°). In contrast, a larger angle deviation was noted (i.e., 2.8°) when the arrow image was employed. This result is consistent with those of oVEMP.

Additionally, she was found to have a mild sensorineural hearing loss at high frequencies bilaterally (Figure 2), with normal tympanometric findings (suggestive of a normal middle ear function). The pure tone audiometry and tympanometry were performed in accordance with the recommended procedures (13, 14), using a two-channel audiometer (GSI 61, Grason-Stadler Inc., USA) and a 226 Hz tympanometer (GSI TympStar Pro, Grason-Stadler Inc., USA), respectively.

Discussion

Due to vestibular dysfunctions, the affected individuals may report symptoms such as imbalance, vertigo, lightheadedness, pre-syncope, and nonspecific dizziness (15). Vertigo ("the spinning sensation") is typically reported by patients with impaired semicircular canals (2, 16). Other subtypes of dizziness are experienced by patients with lesions affecting otolith organs and/or the central vestibular pathways (2, 17). Therefore, comprehensive history taking and specialized assessments are imperative to accurately diagnose vestibular disorders.

In this chapter, the main complaint of the patient was imbalance, and abnormal results were observed in the Fukuda stepping test, oVEMP, and SVV test. As reported elsewhere, the angle rotation of more than 45° in the Fukuda test would suggest the presence of a peripheral vestibular asymmetry

(18, 19). Of note, this bedside test has been reported to have high sensitivity in identifying unilateral vestibular lesions (20, 21). This finding is somewhat consistent with the oVEMP results, which showed that the right ear did not produce any discernible peaks. The oVEMP test has been used commonly to offer insights into the function of the utricle and superior vestibular nerve (22). According to the findings of the oVEMP test, it is probable that there could be a dysfunction in the right utricle.

In the SVV test, the patient was instructed to place the visual images to her "best" vertical position (in the absence of visual reference). Given that the utricle is responsible for detecting gravitational forces, which are integral to the perception of verticality, any deviation from the norm in this function would indicate a potential dysfunction of the utricle (23). As found, she performed normally when the visual image was a solid line (i.e., the angle deviation was within ± 2°). In this regard, the SVV test employing a simple visual image was insensitive for identifying a possible utricular dysfunction in this patient. However, when an arrow pattern was used as the visual image, the SVV result became abnormal (i.e., 2.8°). In a study by Zakaria et al. (11), the normative data (90% range) for the arrow pattern was between -1.80° and 2.33°. The abnormal SVV finding is in fact consistent with the results of the oVEMP and Fukuda stepping tests.

This case report demonstrates that using a complex visual image is more advantageous in the SVV test to achieve an accurate vestibular diagnosis. Having this test in clinical settings is particularly useful if other tests (such as oVEMP) are not available or could not be carried out. Furthermore, the SVV test has several notable advantages, including being simple to administer, quick, and cost-effective (e.g., the "bucket" version is available) (23). In terms of the case management, the patient was scheduled to undergo a specialized vestibular rehabilitation program to treat her imbalance problem. Her progress will be monitored from time to time.

Conclusion

Because there are different subtypes of dizziness, it is important to conduct a thorough examination of the patient's history and perform specialized assessments when dealing with patients with vestibular disorders. Evaluating the function of otolith organs is crucial in addressing symptoms of imbalance. The SVV test employing a complex visual image appears to be a more effective method for identifying vestibular dysfunction. Nevertheless, studies utilizing a large sample size is warranted to support the observation reported in this paper.

Declaration of patient consent

The authors certify that they have obtained the consent form from the patient. In the form, the patient has given her consent for her image and other clinical information to be reported in the journal. The patient understands that her name and initial will not be published, and due efforts will be made to conceal her identity, but anonymity cannot be guaranteed.

References

[1] Horak FB. Postural orientation and equilibrium: what do we need to know about neural control of balance to prevent falls? Age Ageing 2006;35(Suppl 2):ii7-ii11.

[2] Katz J, Marshall C, English K, Hood L, Tillery KL. Handbook of clinical audiology. Philadelphia, PA: Lippincott Williams Wilkins, 2015.

[3] Zuraida Z, Mohd Normani Z, Dinsuhaimi S, Zalina I, Geshina MS. Development of Malay version of vertigo symptom scale (MVVSS) for clinical use. Malaysian J Med Health Sci 2010;6(2):31-9.

[4] Moideen A, Konkimalla A, Tyagi AK, Varshney S, Kumar A, Jat B, et al. Cross-sectional analysis of videonystagmography (VNG) findings in balance disorders. Cureus 2023;15(2):e34795.

[5] George M, Kolethekkat AA, Yoan P, Maire R. Video head impulse test: a comparison and analysis of three recording systems. Indian J Otolaryngol Head Neck Surg 2023;75(1):60-6.

[6] Chen G, Zhang J, Qiao Q, Zhou L, Li Y, Yang J, et al. Advances in dynamic visual acuity test research. Front Neurol 2023;13:1047876.

[7] Zuraida Z, Mohd Normani Z, Din Suhaimi S, Zalina I. Sensitivity and specificity of vestibular evoked myogenic potential elicited by different tone bursts to diagnose peripheral vestibular disordered. Malaysian J Med Health Sci 2014;10(2):9-17.

[8] Zakaria MN, Salim R, Anual MSI, Patuzzi R. The narrowband CE-Chirp stimulus does not necessarily produce more robust cervical vestibular evoked myogenic potential. Ear Hear 2024;45(4):1010-8.

[9] Mat Q, Duterme JP, Tainmont S, Lelubre C, Manto M. Optimizing Ocular Vestibular Evoked Myogenic Potentials With Narrow Band CE-Chirps. Ear Hear 2021;42(5):1373-80.

[10] Akin FW, Murnane OD. Subjective visual vertical test. Semin Hear 2009;30:281-6.

[11] Zakaria MN, Salim R, Tahir A, Zainun Z, Mohd Sakeri NS. The influences of age, gender and geometric pattern of visual image on the verticality perception: A

subjective visual vertical (SVV) study among Malaysian adults. Clin Otolaryngol 2019;44(2):166-71.

[12] Zakaria MN, Tahir A, Zainun Z, Salim R, Mohd Sakeri NS, Abdul Wahat NH. The influence of type of visual image and gender on the perception of horizontality: a subjective visual horizontal (SVH) study. Acta Otolaryngol 2021;141(1):62-5.

[13] Romli M, Wan Mohamad WN, Awang MA, Aw CL, Zakaria MN. The clinical value of bilateral bone conduction testing in hearing diagnosis. Indian J Otol 2020;26(3):182-5.

[14] Lih AC, Zakaria MN, Mohamad RA, Nor Rashid MF. Effects of ethnicity and gender on the middle ear function in Asian adults. Indian J Otol 2017;23(2):94-7.

[15] Post RE, Dickerson LM. Dizziness: a diagnostic approach. Am Fam Physician 2010;82(4):361-8.

[16] Miłoński J, Pietkiewicz P, Bielińska M, Kuśmierczyk K, Olszewski J. The use of videonystagmography head impulse test (VHIT) in the diagnostics of semicircular canal injuries in patients with vertigo. Int J Occup Med Environ Health 2014;27(4):583-90.

[17] Dieterich M. Central vestibular disorders. J Neurol 2007;254(5):559-68.

[18] Fukuda T. The stepping test, two phases of the labyrinthine reflex. Acta Otolaryngol 1959;50:95-108.

[19] Taylan Cebi I, Karatas A. The assessment of fukuda stepping test results in prognosis of benign paroxysmal postural vertigo. Braz J Otorhinolaryngol 2022;88(Suppl 1):S142-6.

[20] Moffat DA, Harries ML, Baguley DM, Hardy DG. Unterberger's stepping test in acoustic neuroma. J Laryngol Otol 1989;103:839-41.

[21] Jacobson GP, Shepard NT. Balance function assessment and management. San Diego, CA: Plural Publishing, 2021.

[22] Weber KP, Rosengren SM. Clinical utility of ocular vestibular-evoked myogenic potentials (oVEMPs). Curr Neurol Neurosci Rep 2015;15(5):22.

[23] Chetana N, Jayesh R. Subjective visual vertical in various vestibular disorders by using a simple bucket test. Indian J Otolaryngol Head Neck Surg 2015;67(2):180-4.

Section four: Acknowledgments

Chapter 23

About the Editors

Mohd N Zakaria, PhD, is currently a Professor and the Chairman of the Audiology Programme, School of Health Sciences, Universiti Sains Malaysia, Malaysia. After obtaining Master of Clinical Audiology and PhD degrees from The University of Western Australia, he returned to Malaysia to serve as a lecturer and a consultant audiologist in a local university. He teaches undergraduate and postgraduate students about various aspects of audiology, otology, neurology and speech sciences. He has authored and co-authored numerous peer-reviewed articles in the fields of diagnostic audiology, auditory physiology, neuroscience, electrophysiology, central auditory disorders, vestibular, tinnitus and biostatistics. He likes to share his knowledge and has presented his research findings in many seminars, conferences and workshops held locally and internationally. His research achievements have been further recognized in which he has been appointed as an Editorial Board Member of many internationally indexed journals and a reviewer for many indexed journals. To keep him further active, Professor Zakaria has supervised over 180 research projects for doctorate, master's and undergraduate degrees. He has also won gold and silver medal awards for his inventions in the field of neuro-otology. Email: mdnorman@usm.my

Joav Merrick, MD, MMedSci, DMSc, born and educated in Denmark, is Professor of Pediatrics, Division of Pediatrics, Hadassah Hebrew University Medical Center, Mt Scopus Campus, Jerusalem, Israel and Kentucky Children's Hospital, University of Kentucky, Lexington, Kentucky United States and professor of public health at the Center for Healthy Development, School of Public Health, Georgia State University, Atlanta, United States, the former medical director of the Health Services, Division for Intellectual and Developmental Disabilities, Ministry of Social Affairs and Social Services, Jerusalem, the founder and director of the National Institute of Child Health

In: Public Health: Audiology Research in Malaysia
Editors: Mohd N. Zakaria and Joav Merrick
ISBN: 979-8-89530-577-5

and Human Development in Israel. Numerous publications in the field of pediatrics, child health and human development, rehabilitation, intellectual disability, disability, health, welfare, abuse, advocacy, quality of life and prevention. Received the Peter Sabroe Child Award for outstanding work on behalf of Danish Children in 1985 and the International LEGO-Prize ("The Children's Nobel Prize") for an extraordinary contribution towards improvement in child welfare and well-being in 1987. In 2017 appointed a Kentucky Colonel by the Commonwealth of Kentucky, the highest honor the governor can bestow to a person. Email: jmerrick@zahav.net.il

Chapter 24

About the Audiology Programme, School of Health Sciences, Universiti Sains Malaysia, Kelantan, Malaysia

Due to specific needs and limited numbers of practising audiologists in Malaysia, the Audiology Programme was established under the School of Health Sciences at the Universiti Sains Malaysia (USM) in the year 2005. Aiming to produce competent graduates to serve disabled populations, the Bachelor in Audiology was introduced. This 4-year course was designed in such a way that the essential aspects (theory, practical and clinical aspects) were sufficiently covered to equip students with knowledge and clinical skills in serving hearing disabled patients of various ages and backgrounds.

Vision and mission

In line with the vision of the School of Health Sciences, USM, the Audiology Programme is committed to be a centre of excellence in the field of audiology towards the wellness of society through intellectual inquiry, creativity, innovation and dissemination of knowledge. To achieve and maintain excellence in these fields, our missions are to produce graduates with a high level of intellectual inquiry and professionalism, develop graduates with a strong sense of ethics and commitment to humanity, and transform knowledge into an instrument for sustainable development and wellness of society.

In: Public Health: Audiology Research in Malaysia
Editors: Mohd N. Zakaria and Joav Merrick
ISBN: 979-8-89530-577-5

Academic activities

The Bachelor in Audiology degree is conducted in a 4-year period. Accredited by the Malaysian Qualification Agency (MQA), this academic programme consists of core, elective and university courses. In order to graduate, students are required to complete 143 credit units with at least 350 clinical hours. Apart from learning the essential theoretical issues in hearing, speech and related disciplines, students are trained to become competent clinicians through extensive clinical placements and teaching. To further enhance the clinical exposure and experience, the Audiology Programme has also established linkages with external agencies and institutions through students' placements in government hospitals, private hospitals, special education schools, hearing aid and implant companies and other universities in Malaysia.

Clinical activities

The Audiology Clinic, USM, is the major centre for clinical teaching, services and research. Both basic and advanced clinical services are offered to suit the needs of patients. Students are attached and supervised by experienced clinicians in these clinics during their clinical years. In the Audiology Clinic, apart from providing basic audiological services (routine audiological assessments, hearing aid fitting/evaluation etc.), specialized services such as for those with tinnitus, balance/vestibular disorders and auditory processing disorder are also offered.

Research activities

Various research projects in the fields of otorhinolaryngology and hearing have been conducted by respective undergraduate, master and PhD candidates. Many of the research findings have been peer-reviewed and published in reputable indexed journals. Furthermore, innovative products for hearing, speech, vestibular and tinnitus assessments and treatments have been developed and validated accordingly to improve the current clinical services, as well as to provide alternative solutions in clinical management.

In particular, for advanced hearing assessments, Malay version of masking level difference (MLD) test, Malay version of binaural fusion test and Malay version of auditory figure ground test have been developed and are available for clinical applications. Currently, a new speech test known as Speech Perception in Echo and Noise Test (SPENT) is being tested for its efficacy and sensitivity among pediatric population. To optimize results when performing auditory electrophysiological tests, custom-build chirp stimuli namely auditory brainstem response Based Experimental chirp (ABE-chirp) and downward narrow-band chirp have been constructed.

These stimuli have been tested for their usefulness among normal and pathological subjects. Moreover, an interactive rehabilitation module, i.e., interactive Computerized Auditory Rehabilitation (i-CARE) has been developed and validated among hearing-impaired children. As revealed by subjective and objective results, this rehabilitation method has been found to be useful in improving specific auditory skills of hearing-impaired children.

To document the effects of tinnitus on patients' daily life activities, a tinnitus questionnaire known as Borang Evaluasi Soalselidik Tinitus (BEST) has been developed and validated to be used among Malay population. This questionnaire has been used by many tinnitus centres in Malaysia. In addition, in order to find optimum treatment for tinnitus, novel spectrally modified stimuli have been studied and proven to be beneficial. These stimuli have been regularly prescribed in specialized tinnitus clinics in Malaysia to provide short-term and long-term relief among tinnitus sufferers.

Balance disorders are common among adults and ongoing research is imperative in search of optimum assessments and treatments. As such, several innovative balance assessment products have been studied and are available for clinical use. Currently, a cost-effective product for assessing the function of vestibular organs is being studied among normal and pathological subjects. To improve the balance function and provide relief from vertigo, Balance Exercise (Bal Ex) products have been developed and validated accordingly. Most of these products are home-based, which are advantageous to both patients and clinicians.

Conclusion

Academic teaching, clinical supervision, clinical services and research are the main activities carried out actively by dedicated clinicians, students, researchers and lecturers in the Audiology Programme, USM. These activities are to be sustained and improved from time to time to maintain the vision and mission of this programme.

Contact

Professor Mohd Normani Zakaria, MClinAud, PhD
Chairman of Audiology Programme, School of Health Sciences,
Universiti Sains Malaysia, Kelantan, Malaysia.
Email: mdnorman@usm.my

Chapter 25

About the National Institute of Child Health and Human Development in Israel

The National Institute of Child Health and Human Development (NICHD) in Israel was established in 1998 as a virtual institute under the auspices of the Medical Director, Ministry of Social Affairs and Social Services in order to function as the research arm for the Office of the Medical Director. In 1998 the National Council for Child Health and Pediatrics, Ministry of Health and in 1999 the Director General and Deputy Director General of the Ministry of Health endorsed the establishment of the NICHD.

Mission

The mission of a National Institute for Child Health and Human Development in Israel is to provide an academic focal point for the scholarly interdisciplinary study of child life, health, public health, welfare, disability, rehabilitation, intellectual disability and related aspects of human development. This mission includes research, teaching, clinical work, information and public service activities in the field of child health and human development.

Service and academic activities

Over the years many activities became focused in the south of Israel due to collaboration with various professionals at the Faculty of Health Sciences (FOHS) at the Ben Gurion University of the Negev (BGU). Since 2000 an affiliation with the Zusman Child Development Center at the Pediatric

In: Public Health: Audiology Research in Malaysia
Editors: Mohd N. Zakaria and Joav Merrick
ISBN: 979-8-89530-577-5

Division of Soroka University Medical Center has resulted in collaboration around the establishment of the Down Syndrome Clinic at that center. In 2002 a full course on "Disability" was established at the Recanati School for Allied Professions in the Community, FOHS, BGU and in 2005 collaboration was started with the Primary Care Unit of the faculty and disability became part of the master of public health course on "Children and society." In the academic year 2005-2006 a one semester course on "Aging with disability" was started as part of the master of science program in gerontology in our collaboration with the Center for Multidisciplinary Research in Aging. In 2010 collaborations with the Division of Pediatrics, Hadassah Hebrew University Medical Center, Jerusalem, Israel around the National Down Syndrome Center and teaching students and residents about intellectual and developmental disabilities as part of their training at this campus.

Research activities

The affiliated staff have over the years published work from projects and research activities in this national and international collaboration. In the year 2000 the International Journal of Adolescent Medicine and Health and in 2005 the International Journal on Disability and Human Development of De Gruyter Publishing House (Berlin and New York) were affiliated with the National Institute of Child Health and Human Development. From 2008 also the International Journal of Child Health and Human Development (Nova Science, New York), the International Journal of Child and Adolescent Health (Nova Science) and the Journal of Pain Management (Nova Science) affiliated and from 2009 the International Public Health Journal (Nova Science) and Journal of Alternative Medicine Research (Nova Science). All peer-reviewed international journals.

National collaborations

Nationally the NICHD works in collaboration with the Faculty of Health Sciences, Ben Gurion University of the Negev; Department of Physical Therapy, Sackler School of Medicine, Tel Aviv University; Autism Center, Assaf HaRofeh Medical Center; National Rett and PKU Centers at Chaim Sheba Medical Center, Tel HaShomer; Department of Physiotherapy, Haifa

University; Department of Education, Bar Ilan University, Ramat Gan, Faculty of Social Sciences and Health Sciences; College of Judea and Samaria in Ariel and in 2011 affiliation with Center for Pediatric Chronic Diseases and National Center for Down Syndrome, Department of Pediatrics, Hadassah Hebrew University Medical Center, Mount Scopus Campus, Jerusalem.

International collaborations

Internationally with the Department of Disability and Human Development, College of Applied Health Sciences, University of Illinois at Chicago; Strong Center for Developmental Disabilities, Golisano Children's Hospital at Strong, University of Rochester School of Medicine and Dentistry, New York; Centre on Intellectual Disabilities, University of Albany, New York; Centre for Chronic Disease Prevention and Control, Health Canada, Ottawa; Chandler Medical Center and Children's Hospital, Kentucky Children's Hospital, Section of Adolescent Medicine, University of Kentucky, Lexington; Chronic Disease Prevention and Control Research Center, Baylor College of Medicine, Houston, Texas; Division of Neuroscience, Department of Psychiatry, Columbia University, New York; Institute for the Study of Disadvantage and Disability, Atlanta; Center for Autism and Related Disorders, Department Psychiatry, Children's Hospital Boston, Boston; Department of Pediatric and Adolescent Medicine, Western Michigan University Homer Stryker MD School of Medicine, Kalamazoo, Michigan, United States; Department of Paediatrics, Child Health and Adolescent Medicine, Children's Hospital at Westmead, Westmead, Australia; International Centre for the Study of Occupational and Mental Health, Düsseldorf, Germany; Centre for Advanced Studies in Nursing, Department of General Practice and Primary Care, University of Aberdeen, Aberdeen, United Kingdom; Quality of Life Research Center, Copenhagen, Denmark; Nordic School of Public Health, Gottenburg, Sweden, Scandinavian Institute of Quality of Working Life, Oslo, Norway; The Department of Applied Social Sciences (APSS) of The Hong Kong Polytechnic University Hong Kong.

Targets

Our focus is on research, international collaborations, clinical work, teaching and policy in health, disability and human development and to establish the NICHD as a permanent institute in Israel in order to conduct model research and policy.

Contact

Professor Joav Merrick, MD, MMedSci, DMSc
Director, National Institute of Child Health and Human Development, Jerusalem, Israel.
Email: jmerrick@zahav.net.il

Section five: Index

Index

A

acoustic, 7, 12, 13, 15, 18, 42, 45, 46, 47, 48, 65, 67, 86, 108, 115, 119, 120, 122, 129, 130, 131, 132, 134, 136, 153, 155, 157, 171, 173, 174, 175, 176, 177, 180, 199, 201, 203, 220
acoustic reflex, 129, 130, 131, 132, 134, 136, 153, 155, 173, 177, 199, 201, 203
age-related, 54
audiology, 3, 4, 5, 6, 8, 9, 17, 26, 38, 48, 55, 56, 57, 59, 60, 61, 78, 82, 87, 93, 98, 103, 127, 135, 136, 147, 153, 154, 158, 163, 168, 171, 176, 177, 181, 185, 202, 203, 205, 207, 211, 213, 219, 223, 225, 226, 227, 228
audiometric, 28, 71, 184, 201, 202, 205, 206, 207, 209, 210, 211
auditory brainstem response (ABR), 5, 6, 7, 12, 17, 20, 21, 23, 24, 26, 27, 43, 49, 63, 66, 67, 68, 69, 71, 72, 77, 83, 87, 94, 104, 121, 122, 123, 124, 125, 126, 127, 128, 131, 133, 134, 135, 136, 137, 141, 147, 157, 158, 185, 211, 227
auditory processing disorder(s) (APD), 11, 13, 14, 15, 16, 17, 18, 127, 226
auditory steady state response (ASSR), 12, 17, 19, 20, 21, 22, 23, 24, 25, 26, 27, 28, 43, 49, 83, 104, 135, 211

B

baby(ies), 67, 135, 147, 189, 190, 193, 211
behavioural, 19, 20, 21, 22, 23, 24, 25, 65, 142, 145, 146, 180, 181, 184, 185, 187
behavioural hearing thresholds, 19, 21, 22
bone conduction (BC), 6, 17, 25, 26, 38, 39, 48, 59, 69, 83, 94, 95, 96, 97, 98, 101, 102, 104, 128, 135, 137, 146, 147, 151, 152, 156, 158, 163, 168, 171, 172, 173, 174, 175, 176, 177, 185, 186, 195, 197, 198, 199, 200, 201, 202, 203, 205, 206, 207, 210, 220
brainstem, 12, 22, 23, 28, 42, 49, 63, 64, 66, 67, 68, 71, 72, 83, 94, 121, 122, 123, 126, 127, 128, 129, 131, 133, 134, 136, 211

C

central auditory nervous system (CANS), 11, 12, 13, 64
cervical, 75, 76, 79, 83, 85, 86, 89, 90, 93, 94, 214, 219
children, 3, 6, 8, 11, 12, 13, 14, 15, 16, 17, 18, 19, 22, 23, 25, 26, 27, 31, 32, 33, 35, 36, 37, 38, 39, 40, 41, 42, 43, 44, 45, 47, 48, 49, 50, 54, 60, 67, 71, 104, 120, 127, 136, 139, 141, 142, 143, 144, 145, 146, 147, 148, 152, 162, 166, 167, 168, 169, 179, 180, 181, 183, 184, 186, 189, 190, 194, 195, 211, 223, 227, 230, 231
chirp, 5, 7, 20, 23, 28, 75, 77, 78, 79, 80, 81, 82, 83, 85, 87, 88, 89, 90, 91, 92, 93, 94, 103, 219, 227
cochlear implant(s) (CIs), 6, 7, 37, 39, 41, 42, 45, 48, 49, 50, 51, 56, 140, 141, 147, 148, 163, 166, 169, 179, 180, 184, 185, 186, 187
cognitive behavioural therapy, 54, 57, 58, 65

communication(s), 12, 13, 19, 20, 55, 56, 60, 64, 76, 96, 119, 154, 198, 205
cortical auditory evoked potential (CAEP), 6, 8, 12, 17, 21, 26, 31, 32, 33, 35, 36, 37, 38, 39, 40, 41, 43, 44, 45, 46, 47, 48, 49, 50, 51, 71, 127, 136, 139, 140, 141, 142, 143, 144, 145, 147, 161, 162, 164, 165, 166, 167, 168, 169, 179, 181, 182, 183, 184, 185, 186
cross-hearing, 96, 151, 152, 153, 155, 156, 157

D

device(s), 21, 23, 32, 33, 35, 41, 42, 43, 45, 47, 48, 78, 80, 88, 123, 140, 142, 153, 164, 167, 179, 180, 181, 182, 183, 184, 216
diagnosing, 11, 16, 71, 95, 130, 171, 174, 197, 199

E

earphones, 75, 78, 88, 95, 96, 97, 98, 99, 100, 101, 102, 103, 163, 175
earwax blockage, 54
electrode montage, 161, 163, 165, 166, 167
environment(s), 11, 12, 13, 14, 16, 18, 47, 55, 60, 76, 122, 130, 154, 172, 199

F

frequency range(s), 45, 78, 85, 87, 88, 89, 91, 92
frequency(ies), 17, 20, 21, 22, 23, 25, 26, 27, 28, 36, 39, 44, 45, 47, 49, 64, 72, 77, 78, 83, 85, 86, 87, 88, 89, 91, 92, 93, 96, 97, 98, 99, 100, 101, 102, 103, 104, 106, 112, 115, 120, 129, 131, 132, 133, 134, 135, 136, 142, 147, 153, 155, 156, 163, 168, 171, 172, 173, 174, 175, 176, 197, 198, 199, 200, 201, 202, 203, 206, 207, 208, 209, 211, 217

G

gender, 7, 17, 26, 39, 49, 59, 67, 69, 71, 82, 83, 93, 103, 104, 106, 107, 108, 112, 113, 115, 117, 118, 120, 127, 128, 135, 136, 137, 143, 147, 158, 159, 168, 177, 185, 195, 203, 210, 211, 219, 220
glottal area waveform (GAW), 105, 106, 115, 120
glottis, 110, 111, 112, 113, 114, 116, 117, 119

H

headphones, 16, 21, 95, 96, 97, 98, 99, 100, 101, 102, 103, 152, 153, 156
healthcare, 3, 4, 6, 20, 24, 25, 28, 54, 57, 58, 60, 61, 65, 130, 140, 151, 172
hearing aid (HA), 6, 25, 31, 32, 33, 35, 36, 37, 38, 39, 42, 45, 50, 54, 56, 59, 60, 61, 65, 70, 139, 140, 141, 142, 144, 145, 147, 148, 161, 162, 163, 164, 166, 168, 181, 183, 198, 209, 213, 226
hearing loss, 4, 5, 8, 12, 15, 17, 19, 20, 22, 23, 25, 26, 27, 28, 32, 35, 39, 40, 42, 45, 50, 54, 55, 58, 59, 60, 65, 68, 69, 70, 71, 95, 96, 97, 102, 104, 127, 140, 142, 146, 147, 152, 156, 157, 162, 163, 171, 172, 173, 174, 175, 180, 181, 183, 184, 186, 189, 195, 198, 199, 200, 201, 203, 205, 206, 207, 208, 209, 211
hearing-impaired, 18, 20, 23, 25, 26, 31, 32, 33, 35, 36, 37, 38, 42, 48, 64, 97, 102, 139, 144, 163, 166, 167, 183, 184, 227

L

language, 5, 12, 13, 16, 17, 18, 19, 25, 32, 36, 37, 40, 42, 43, 48, 60, 61, 65, 108, 120, 142, 145, 147, 162, 166, 167, 180, 181, 183, 184, 213
laryngeal high-speed videoendoscopy (LHSV), 105, 106, 107, 108, 109, 117, 118, 119, 120

listening, 11, 12, 13, 14, 15, 16, 18, 35, 44, 47, 76, 122, 141, 142, 167, 172
loud noises, 54, 199, 201

M

machine learning, 20, 24, 28, 29
Malaysia, 3, 4, 5, 6, 7, 8, 11, 16, 17, 18, 19, 25, 31, 41, 53, 59, 61, 63, 69, 70, 75, 82, 85, 92, 94, 95, 103, 105, 119, 121, 129, 135, 139, 146, 151, 161, 171, 176, 179, 189, 197, 202, 205, 210, 213, 223, 225, 226, 227, 228
mechanism(s), 63, 64, 67, 68, 69, 130, 156, 159, 198
medication(s), 54, 64, 140, 198, 199

N

neural, 22, 24, 33, 41, 43, 44, 63, 67, 68, 87, 139, 144, 145, 167, 168, 184, 198, 219
noise, 7, 12, 13, 14, 15, 16, 18, 21, 22, 28, 64, 65, 66, 71, 97, 98, 99, 100, 102, 121, 122, 123, 124, 125, 126, 153, 154, 156, 209, 227
normal speakers, 105, 106, 108, 115, 116, 118, 120
Nyquist plots, 106, 107, 113, 116, 117

P

paediatric, 7, 20, 35, 38, 41, 146, 162, 180, 181, 186, 187, 195
patient(s), 4, 5, 6, 7, 17, 19, 20, 21, 23, 26, 38, 42, 45, 53, 54, 55, 56, 57, 58, 59, 60, 64, 65, 66, 67, 68, 69, 70, 71, 72, 76, 81, 82, 86, 93, 96, 97, 102, 104, 122, 123, 126, 128, 129, 130, 131, 133, 134, 135, 136, 137, 140, 146, 147, 153, 154, 155, 156, 157, 158, 159, 167, 168, 174, 175, 176, 181, 182, 183, 184, 185, 187, 190, 194, 195, 197, 199, 200, 201, 202, 203, 206, 207, 208, 209, 210, 211, 213, 215, 216, 217, 218, 219, 220, 225, 226, 227
perception, 6, 11, 12, 14, 15, 16, 36, 39, 41, 43, 47, 49, 50, 54, 64, 65, 66, 68, 82, 93, 103, 169, 183, 186, 206, 207, 217, 218, 219, 220, 227
performance(s), 12, 15, 18, 19, 20, 22, 32, 36, 37, 42, 43, 49, 60, 127, 135, 147, 166, 176, 186, 203, 210
physiological, 63, 67, 69, 71, 126, 168
pure tone audiometry (PTA), 5, 12, 13, 17, 20, 23, 25, 28, 38, 77, 87, 95, 96, 97, 98, 99, 101, 103, 104, 123, 131, 135, 141, 147, 151, 152, 153, 154, 155, 156, 157, 158, 159, 168, 171, 172, 173, 174, 175, 176, 198, 199, 200, 202, 205, 206, 207, 208, 209, 210, 216, 217

R

recorded, 21, 22, 27, 32, 44, 45, 47, 66, 67, 75, 77, 78, 79, 80, 81, 85, 109, 125, 133, 141, 142, 165, 183, 186
reflex, 26, 43, 48, 129, 130, 131, 134, 136, 157, 173, 177, 180, 181, 182, 185, 186, 200, 203, 215, 220
reverberant, 11, 14, 15, 16, 18
ringing sound in the ear, 53

S

schizophrenia, 5, 7, 17, 26, 38, 59, 69, 104, 123, 126, 128, 129, 130, 131, 132, 133, 134, 136, 137, 146, 147, 158, 159, 168, 176, 185, 202, 210
sensorineural acuity level (SAL), 95, 97, 98, 99, 101, 102, 103, 104
sensorineural hearing loss (SNHL), 22, 28, 31, 32, 37, 39, 42, 72, 96, 101, 139, 140, 141, 142, 143, 144, 145, 148, 153, 161, 163, 169, 172, 173, 175, 176, 179, 181, 189, 195, 197, 198, 199, 200, 201, 206, 207, 208, 211, 217
sound(s), 6, 7, 12, 14, 15, 20, 21, 24, 25, 26, 32, 33, 36, 38, 39, 42, 43, 44, 48, 49, 54, 55, 59, 63, 64, 65, 66, 69, 70, 71, 93, 98, 119, 122, 124, 128, 130, 135, 141,

146, 154, 156, 158, 164, 166, 168, 172, 174, 176, 180, 181, 199, 202, 209, 210
speech, 5, 6, 7, 11, 12, 13, 14, 15, 16, 17, 18, 19, 25, 26, 31, 32, 36, 38, 39, 41, 42, 43, 44, 45, 47, 48, 49, 50, 60, 61, 70, 71, 83, 104, 108, 119, 120, 121, 122, 127, 128, 130, 135, 139, 140, 141, 142, 145, 147, 158, 161, 163, 164, 165, 166, 167, 169, 179, 180, 181, 183, 184, 185, 186, 211, 213, 223, 226, 227
stimulation(s), 25, 42, 43, 44, 45, 46, 47, 48, 50, 66, 83, 94, 121, 122, 123, 124, 125, 126, 128, 132, 134, 136, 181, 186
subjective visual vertical (SVV), 82, 93, 103, 213, 214, 216, 217, 218, 219, 220

T

teleaudiology, 6, 8, 53, 55, 56, 57, 58, 60, 61
therapeutic, 3
tinnitus, 4, 5, 7, 26, 38, 53, 54, 55, 56, 57, 58, 59, 60, 61, 62, 63, 64, 65, 66, 67, 68, 69, 70, 71, 72, 128, 135, 137, 146, 153, 154, 157, 158, 168, 172, 175, 176, 198, 199, 202, 210, 223, 226, 227
tone burst stimuli, 75, 77, 78, 79, 80
transducer, 95, 96, 98, 100, 101, 102, 103, 176, 203
treatment(s), 5, 16, 25, 26, 32, 42, 54, 57, 63, 65, 66, 70, 76, 96, 128, 130, 140, 147, 172, 174, 180, 183, 189, 190, 193, 194, 198, 206, 208, 214, 226, 227
tuning fork, 205, 206, 207, 209, 211

U

user(s), 7, 33, 37, 39, 41, 45, 46, 47, 48, 50, 51, 56, 62, 116, 140, 141, 144, 161, 166, 167, 169, 184, 185, 186, 187

V

vestibular, 4, 5, 6, 7, 28, 75, 76, 78, 79, 81, 82, 83, 85, 86, 87, 88, 89, 90, 92, 93, 94, 96, 103, 104, 123, 127, 135, 176, 186, 202, 210, 213, 214, 215, 217, 218, 219, 220, 223, 226, 227
vestibular evoked myogenic potential (VEMP), 28, 75, 76, 77, 79, 82, 83, 85, 86, 89, 90, 93, 94, 103, 214, 219
vibratory, 105, 106, 107, 116, 118, 119, 120
videoendoscopy, 105, 119, 120
visual image, 82, 93, 103, 213, 215, 216, 217, 218, 219, 220
vocal, 105, 106, 108, 109, 112, 115, 116, 118, 119, 120
voiceless, 140, 142

W

waveform(s), 21, 23, 27, 32, 35, 36, 43, 44, 45, 47, 48, 50, 67, 75, 76, 77, 78, 79, 81, 87, 88, 89, 91, 92, 122, 124, 125, 126, 133, 139, 141, 144, 145, 161, 162, 165, 166, 180, 182, 183, 184, 217
Weber test, 205, 206, 207, 209, 210, 211
well-being, 53, 55, 64, 224